Obesity and Cardiovascular Disease

Obesity and Cardiovascular Disease

Gianluca Iacobellis MD PhD

Associate Professor of Endocrinology,
Department of Medicine, McMaster University,
Hamilton, Ontario, Canada

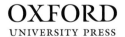

OXFORD
UNIVERSITY PRESS

OXFORD
UNIVERSITY PRESS

Great Clarendon Street, Oxford OX2 6DP

Oxford University Press is a department of the University of Oxford.
It furthers the University's objective of excellence in research, scholarship,
and education by publishing worldwide in

Oxford New York

Auckland Cape Town Dar es Salaam Hong Kong Karachi
Kuala Lumpur Madrid Melbourne Mexico City Nairobi
New Delhi Shanghai Taipei Toronto

With offices in

Argentina Austria Brazil Chile Czech Republic France Greece
Guatemala Hungary Italy Japan Poland Portugal Singapore
South Korea Switzerland Thailand Turkey Ukraine Vietnam

Oxford is a registered trade mark of Oxford University Press
in the UK and in certain other countries

Published in the United States
by Oxford University Press Inc., New York

© Oxford University Press, 2009

British Library Cataloguing in Publication Data

Data available

Library of Congress Cataloging in Publication Data
Iacobellis, Gianluca.
 Obesity and cardiovascular disease / Gianluca Iacobellis.
   p. ; cm.
 Includes bibliographical references and index.
 ISBN 978-0-19-954932-0 (pbk.)
 1. Obesity—Complications. 2. Cardiovascular system—Diseases—Risk factors.
 I. Title.
 [DNLM: 1. Obesity—complications. 2. Cardiovascular Diseases—etiology.
WD 210 I11o 2009]
 RC628.I23 2009
 616.3'98—dc22

Typeset in Minion by Cepha Imaging Private Ltd., Bangalore, India
Printed in Great Britain
on acid-free paper by the
MPG Books Group, Bodmin and King's Lynn

ISBN 978-0-19-954932-0 (Pbk.)

10 9 8 7 6 5 4 3 2 1

Author biography

Professor Gianluca Iacobellis is currently Associate Professor of Endocrinology, Department of Medicine, McMaster University, Hamilton, Ontario, Canada; Director of Bariatric Endocrinology; Consultant Endocrinologist at the Bariatric Centre of Excellence, Department of Medicine, St. Joseph's Hospital, Hamilton, Ontario, Canada.

Prof. Iacobellis obtained his Medical Doctor (MD) degree *cum laude* in 1994, at the University of Roma, La Sapienza, Italy; he was a Research Fellow at the Centrum for Metabolism & Endocrinology, Karolinska University, Stockholm, Sweden, in 1999; a Specialist in Diabetology, Endocrinology, and Metabolic Disorders in 2000; and did his PhD in Endocrinology, Metabolic and Cardiovascular Disorders at the University of Roma, La Sapienza, in 2004. Dr Iacobellis was invited to be a Post-doctoral Clinical Research Fellow at the Center for Human Nutrition, Southwestern Medical Center, Dallas, Texas, USA, from 2004 to 2005. He was a Clinical Research Fellow in the Cardiovascular Obesity Research & Management and Bariatric Clinic, Hamilton Health Sciences, McMaster University, Hamilton, Ontario, Canada, from 2005 to 2006.

Prof. Iacobellis has authored and co-authored more than 60 peer-reviewed papers and ten textbooks. His research and clinical interest is mainly focused on cardiovascular risk in obesity and metabolic syndrome. He pioneered and developed echocardiographic epicardial fat quantification as a practical and reliable marker of visceral adiposity and as a therapeutic target. He has lectured widely on obesity and cardiovascular disease, and is currently the principal investigator and co-investigator of several clinical trials. Dr Iacobellis recently started, as editor-in-chief, a new scientific journal, *Journal of EndoCardiology*, published by Nova Science Publishers, New York, USA.

Foreword

Obesity has now overtaken smoking as the principal risk factor for cardiovascular disease in most Western societies. The root causes of the obesity epidemic are complex; despite major efforts, the global increase in obesity rates continues to rise and childhood obesity is rampant.

Not only does obesity contribute to cardiovascular disease as a risk factor, but it is now also evident that adipose tissue itself produces a vast array of molecules (adipokines) that directly influence cardiovascular and metabolic function. Thus, for example, the adipose-tissue-derived factor leptin not only plays an important role in the regulation of energy homeostasis, but also increases sympathetic nerve activity, thereby increasing cardiac output and promoting volume retention. Other adipose-tissue-derived factors such as visfatin, resistin, and adiponectin are likewise recognized to play important roles in the obesity-related pathologies of the cardiovascular system.

Despite the recognition that obesity is an important mediator of cardiovascular risk, our ability to clinically address and manage obesity remains limited. Short of bariatric surgery, we still lack hard outcome data on the effects of weight loss on cardiovascular mortality. Nevertheless, current behavioral and medical approaches to obesity management do have significant beneficial effects on other cardiovascular risk factors and it appears prudent that weight loss is recommended as a first-line treatment to anyone in whom excess weight appears to be contributing to hypertension, dysplipidemia, or type 2 diabetes mellitus.

For clinicians dealing with obesity-related health problems, this compendium on obesity and cardiovascular disease could not come at a better time. Not only has Prof. Iacobellis himself made significant research contributions to the field (for example, on the role of epicardial fat), but he has succeeded in summarizing for the busy clinician the major discoveries, treatments, and controversies in obesity-related cardiovascular disease. His particular expertise in cardiac imaging is well reflected in these pages—his own experience as a practicing physician and obesity researcher makes the book relevant to both the practitioner and the student of this topic.

Given the importance of obesity as a key determinant of cardiovascular disease, it is expected that this field will continue developing at a rapid pace. Nevertheless, the many chapters of this book will provide a solid foundation to anyone looking for a current update on how obesity affects cardiovascular health and what to do about it.

I am certain that the readers of this book will come away with a much broader appreciation of the complex nature of obesity and its manifold impact on cardiovascular and metabolic disease. This appreciation is the first step towards ultimately reducing the burden of obesity-related cardiovascular disease on our patients.

Arya M Sharma

MD/PhD
FRCPC Professor and Chair in
Obesity Research and Management
University of Alberta
Edmonton
Canada

Contents

Contributors

Navneet Singh
Bachelor Health Sciences
Honours, McMaster University,
Hamilton, ON, Canada
Senior Medical Student at the
University of Toronto, ON,
Canada

Dennis Wei
Bachelor Life Sciences Honours,
Queen's University Kingston,
ON, Canada
Biomedical Communications
Fellow at University of Toronto,
ON, Canada

Abbreviations

ACE	angiotensin-converting enzyme		DTE	deceleration time of early diastolic mitral flow
AF	atrial fibrillation		DVT	deep vein thrombosis
apo	apolipoprotein		ECG	electrocardiogram
ARB	angiotensin II type 1 receptor blocker		EF	ejection fraction
AT_1	angiotensin II type 1		Es	early peak diastolic mitral annulus velocity
ATP III	Adult Treatment Panel III		ET	ejection time
BIA	bioelectrical impedance		ET-1	endothelin-1
BMI	body mass index		FDA	US Food and Drug Administration
BNP	B-type natriuretic peptide		FFM	fat-free mass
BSA	body surface area		FM	fat mass
CB-1	endocannabinoid receptor 1		GLP-1	glucagon-like peptide-1
CCHS	Canadian Community Health Survey		HbA1c	glycosylated hemoglobin
CDC	Centers for Disease Control and Prevention		HDL	high-density lipoprotein
cESS	circumferential end-systolic stress		HOMA-IR	homeostasis model assessment of insulin resistance
CI	confidence interval		HRV	heart rate variability
c IMT	carotid intima–media thickness		HU	Hounsfield unit
cMWS	circumferential mid-wall shortening		IBS	integrated backscatter
			ICAM-1	intercellular adhesion molecule-1
CRP	C-reactive protein		IFG	impaired fasting glucose
CT	computed tomography		IGT	impaired glucose tolerance
CTCA	computed tomography coronary angiography		IL-6	interleukin-6
DBP	diastolic blood pressure		INR	international normalized ratio
DEXA	dual-energy X-ray absorptiometry		IOTF	International Obesity Task Force
DPP4	dipeptidyl peptidase-4		IVCT	isovolumic contraction time

IVRT	isovolumic relaxation time		1H-MRS	proton magnetic resonance spectroscopy
IVUS	intravascular ultrasound		MWS	mid-wall shortening
JNC	Joint National Committee on Prevention, Detection, Evaluation, and Treatment of High Blood Pressure		NGF	nerve growth factor
			NHANES	National Health and Examination Survey
			NO	nitric oxide
			NT-proBNP	N-terminal fragment of B-type natriuretic peptide
LA	left atrium			
LCD	low-calorie diet		OGTT	oral glucose tolerance test
LDL	low-density lipoprotein			
LMWH	low-molecular-weight heparin		OSA	obstructive sleep apnea
			PAI-1	plasminogen activator inhibitor-1
LRYGB	laparoscopic Roux-en-Y gastric bypass			
			PET	positron emission tomography
LSG	laparoscopic sleeve gastrectomy		PWS	posterior wall thickness
LV	left ventricle			
LVEDD	left ventricle end-diastolic diameter		PWTD	posterior wall thickness in diastole
			QTc	QT-corrected
LVEDV	left ventricle end-diastolic volume		RAS	rennin–angiotensin system
LVESD	left ventricle end-systolic diameter		RBP4	retinol-binding protein 4
LVIDD	left ventricular internal diameter in diastole		RV	right ventricle
			RVEDD	right ventricle end-diastolic diameter
LVH	left ventricle hypertrophy			
			RVESD	right ventricle end-systolic diameter
LVM	left ventricle mass			
MCP-1	monocyte chemoattractant protein-1		RWT	relative wall thickness
			SAECG	small high-frequency electrocardiogram potentials
MDCT	multi-detector computed tomography			
			SBP	systolic blood pressure
mESS	meridional end-systolic stress		SNS	sympathetic nervous system
MHO	metabolically healthy but obese		SPET	single-photon emission computed tomography
MPI	myocardial performance index			
			SRI	strain rate imaging
			TDI	tissue Doppler imaging
MRI	magnetic resonance imaging		TNF-α	tumor necrosis factor-α

VCAM-1	vascular cell adhesion molecule-1	WHO	World Health Organization
VLCD	very-low-calorie diet	WHR	waist-to-hip ratio
VLDL	very-low-density lipoprotein		

Chapter 1

Introduction: redefinition of the relationship between obesity and the cardiovascular system

The fact that excess fat can be an unfavorable medical condition has been noted since earliest times. In fact, in 400 BC, Hippocrates astutely observed that '*sudden death is more common in those who are naturally fat than in the lean*'.

Historically, obese individuals, that is subjects with excess fat accumulation, have been considered more prone to develop cardiovascular disease than individuals with normal body weight. Although this concept remains true, the results of recent research indicate that the relationship between obesity and cardiometabolic diseases should be profoundly revised and reconsidered. The role of excess adiposity in cardiovascular diseases continues to be the subject of debate.

Individuals who are obese are undoubtedly at higher risk of developing hypertension, atherosclerosis, atrial fibrillation, diabetes, peripheral venous disease, and obstructive sleep apnea when compared with individuals who are of normal weight. However, whether an obese individual develops myocardial infarction or heart failure as a result of the co-occurrence of these co-morbidities or as a result of obesity alone is less clear. In fact, although obesity is still a major cardiovascular risk factor, growing evidence shows that obesity is not always related to an unfavorable cardiometabolic profile or to poor cardiac outcome. Whilst the majority of obese individuals have complications, or are at high risk of developing complications, a good number of obese subjects are resistant to the development of adiposity-associated cardiometabolic abnormalities. Obesity-related complications increase the risk of cardiovascular diseases, whereas excess fat by itself and therefore in the absence of co-morbidities (known as uncomplicated metabolically healthy obesity) may lead only to adaptive cardiac morphological and functional changes. The reasons for this common but still underestimated finding are still partially unclear. Subjects who present this protective obesity phenotype are usually young and with more subcutaneous, peripheral adiposity. Genetic, ethnic, environmental, and lifestyle factors are also implicated. These findings underscore the need for further research into the physiological mechanisms underlying the relationship between obesity and cardiovascular diseases.

In addition, obesity seems paradoxically to provide a better outcome and prognosis in subjects who suffer heart failure or undergo cardiac procedures. Several possible mechanisms have been evoked to explain this interesting phenomenon.

The more recently determined and now well-established role of adipose tissue is another good reason to reconsider the relationship between obesity and the heart from a different perspective. Adipose tissue is the new actor on the stage of cardiovascular risk factors.

The reason for the growing scientific and clinical interest in fat is the now widely accepted acknowledgement that adipose tissue is not a silent organ, but is an active source of multiple bioactive cytokines called adipokines. The adipocyte, a mini-organ within this neglected organ, provides output (adipokines) and accepts input via nuclear receptors. Adipose tissue communicates with almost all other organs through endocrine, paracrine, and autocrine interactions. Hence, both systemic and local regulation of the function and morphology of internal organs, including the heart and circulatory system, have recently been attributed to adipose tissue. Fat tissue is also a potentially important responder, due to the presence of multiple receptors that can be modulated, stimulated, or inhibited by drugs with different mechanisms of action and therapeutic purposes. Of additional note is the fact that adipose tissue can now be clinically measured and quantified by simple, accurate, and reliable diagnostic tools. Both biological and clinical characteristics of adipose tissue seem to warrant the successful development of new therapeutic strategies.

The concept and importance of the proximity of adipose tissue to the organs is also intriguing. Intuitively, visceral adipose tissue, that is the fat depots that surround the internal organs, is considered the major cardiovascular risk factor and the most desirable therapeutic target, and great interest has recently been focused on visceral adiposity. The evidence supporting visceral adiposity as an independent cardiometabolic risk factor is robust, with a body of studies suggesting that increased visceral fat plays a significant role in the development of cardiovascular abnormalities.

The scientific community is almost univocal in considering visceral fat to be a greater independent cardiometabolic risk factor than overall obesity. This finding may explain the existence of metabolically healthy but obese subjects, and the different outcomes between subjects with different obesity phenotypes.

The changes in the relationship between obesity and cardiovascular risk, highlighted in this book, relate to the importance of regional fat distribution rather than overall increased adiposity. Subjects with visceral fat accumulation are more prone to, and at higher risk of, cardiovascular diseases than individuals with prevalent peripheral adiposity. This seems to be independent of the body mass index (BMI), and so is independent of obesity. This robust scientific, epidemiological, and clinical evidence has led to profound criticisms of the BMI-based definition and classification of obesity, and to a compelling need for accurate and reliable anthropometric or imaging markers of regional fat distribution. In addition, obesity-related cardiovascular risk varies significantly with ethnicity, age, gender, and dietary habit.

It is intuitive that we should discuss adiposity-related cardiovascular diseases rather than obesity and cardiovascular diseases. We have learned that obesity or, rather, adiposity by itself is not necessarily always associated with cardiovascular disease. Moreover, we should discriminate between visceral and subcutaneous adiposity when we are approaching and managing a subject who can no longer simply be defined as 'obese'. Very recent findings seem to indicate that, even in a clinical setting, our attention should be focused on visceral fat as a major and independent cardiovascular risk factor. It is possible that intracellular fat, that is fat inside the organs, will be a future target.

To date, no well-established diagnostic and therapeutic guidelines for the management and treatment of subjects with excess visceral adiposity have been proposed. Moreover, some aspects remain controversial and contradictory. Some specific recommendations for treating obese subjects or individuals with excess visceral fat accumulation are under development and will be discussed in this book. Whether or not pharmaceutical dosage should be adjusted in obese subjects remains an open and unresolved question. In contrast, treatment of acute cardiovascular events does not differ substantially between obese and normal weight patients. Hence, general recommendations and guidelines for the treatment and management of acute cardiovascular events will apply equally to obese subjects and therefore are not generally described in this book. Technical issues that may occur when performing diagnostic or therapeutic procedures in severely obese subjects will be addressed and discussed.

The reader or clinician who uses this book should thus consider the profound changes and revision of the relationship of obesity with cardiovascular diseases.

Chapter 2

Definition, classification, phenotypes, and epidemiology of obesity

Definition of obesity

Obesity can be defined as an excess of body fat accumulation or adiposity, with multiple organ-specific adaptive or maladaptive consequences. Energy imbalance or a chronic state of positive caloric balance is implicated as the cause of obesity. Adipose cells increase in both size and number. Specific etiological mechanistic interactions affecting energy balance are complex, often including not only biological but also non-biological influences such as socioeconomic conditions and policies. Obesity can be associated with enhanced risk of morbidity and mortality.

Classification of obesity

The World Health Organization (WHO) has set out international guidelines for the classification of weight based on body mass index (BMI), as shown in Table 2.1, that are endorsed by Health Canada and the National Institutes of Health. BMI, the most widely used measure of obesity, is a measure of body fatness based on height and weight. BMI is calculated by dividing the patient's weight in kilograms by their height in meters squared (kg/m^2).

Although this system is still accepted and used worldwide, BMI-based obesity classification has recently been criticized. A more comprehensive obesity classification based also on regional fat distribution and ethnicity has recently been proposed. The advantages and disadvantages of different markers and classifications of obesity are discussed in detail in Chapter 5.

Table 2.1 Obesity classification according to BMI

Classification	BMI category (kg/m^2)
Underweight	<18.5
Normal weight	18.5–24.9
Overweight	25.0–29.9
Obese class I	30.0–34.9
Obese class II	35.0–39.9
Obese class III	≥40.0

Obesity phenotypes

Abdominal adiposity

Adiposity of the abdomen region is referred to as abdominal or central obesity (Figure 2.1). Abdominal obesity potentially results from two stores of fat tissue: subcutaneous and visceral. However, visceral fat is the most predominant adipose tissue depot in subjects with pure

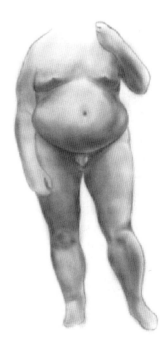

Fig. 2.1 Abdominal obesity phenotype.

abdominal obesity. Individuals with this phenotype present the highest cardiovascular risk. The abdominal obesity phenotype is most commonly observed in Europeans and South Asians. Men are more likely to have a waist distribution of fat compared with women.

Upper truncal adiposity

Adiposity of the thorax is referred to as upper truncal fat. As in subjects with abdominal adiposity, upper truncal fat is composed of both subcutaneous and visceral fat. However, the visceral fat is usually considered the main component of upper truncal fat, as little subcutaneous fat accumulates on the thorax. Those prone to intra-abdominal fat are prone to truncal fat accumulation.

Peripheral adiposity

A peripheral distribution of adiposity is characterized by increase fat in the gluteal region and the upper legs as depicted in Figure 2.2.

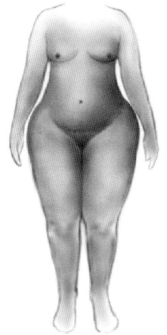

Fig. 2.2 Peripheral obesity phenotype.

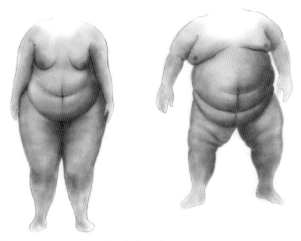

Fig. 2.3 Mixed central–peripheral phenotype.

Women are more likely to have a peripheral distribution of fat than men. This body fat distribution is found most commonly in African-Americans.

Mixed central–peripheral adiposity

A mixed central–peripheral phenotype is characterized by an overall increase in fat accumulation across all body compartments. As shown in Figure 2.3, severely obese women and men (BMI >40 kg/m^2) may both present with this phenotype.

Epidemiology

World prevalence

Worldwide, more than 1.1 billion adults and 10% of children are currently classified as overweight or obese. At least 312 million of these persons are obese. Additionally, as lower cut-off points for obesity for various ethnicities are increasingly recognized (see below), the number of obese individuals increases to 1.7 billion. At all ages and throughout the world, women, due to biological reasons, are generally found to have higher mean BMI values and higher rates of obesity than men.

Childhood obesity

The International Obesity Task Force (IOTF) estimates that approximately 155 million or 10% of school-age children worldwide are classified as overweight. Approximately 30–45 million of these children are estimated to be obese. The IOTF estimates that 2–3% of the world's children between the ages of 5 and 17 are obese. Additionally, for children under the age of 5, approximately 22 million more are at least overweight, with 17 million of them located in developing countries. Within most developing countries, childhood obesity is generally more prevalent among wealthier families. Within developed countries, however, obesity is predominant in lower-income families.

Ethnicity

The IOTF estimates that at least 1.1 billion adults are presently overweight, including 312 million who are obese. However, with the reduction in the Asian BMI criteria of overweight to a cut-off value of 23 kg/m^2, the number of overweight adults worldwide increases to 1.7 billion. Optimum waist circumferences are also lower for Asians: 90 and 80 cm for Asian men and women, respectively, compared with the suggested criteria of 102 and 88 cm for white men and women, respectively. These data have now been incorporated into new proposals by the International Diabetes Federation on the metabolic syndrome with one distinction: the limits for Europid, as distinct from American, white people are 94 cm for men and 80 cm for women. These values and the limits for Japanese, Chinese, and other ethnic groups are based on different criteria and estimates.

Distribution of obesity in North America, Europe, and Asia

USA

Adult obesity More than 72 million Americans are obese or have a BMI ≥30 kg/m^2. According to the National Health and Nutrition Examination Survey (NHANES), 33.5% of male adults and 35.3% of female adults were obese in 2005–2006. The prevalence of obesity is greater in the 40–59 year age group (41.1%) compared with those who are 20–39 (28.1%) or over 60 years (32.2%). Obesity rates in America

have increased steadily since the 1976–1980 survey period. Obesity
rates more than doubled between 1980 and 2004. However, a recent
Centers for Disease Control and Prevention (CDC) study indicated
that the rise is leveling off, as no significant increase was seen for
2003–2004 or 2005–2006. Only a small increase of approximately 2%
in both men and women was noted. There has been a change in the
distribution of BMI since the 1976–1980 period, resulting in a much
heavier adult population today. Racial and ethnic obesity disparities
exist for women but not for men. Approximately 53% of non-
Hispanic black women and 52% of Mexican-American women in the
40–59 year age category were obese compared with 39% of Caucasian
women. Figure 2.4 illustrates the variation in the rise of prevalence of
obesity by individual states. According to the CDC's Behavioral Risk

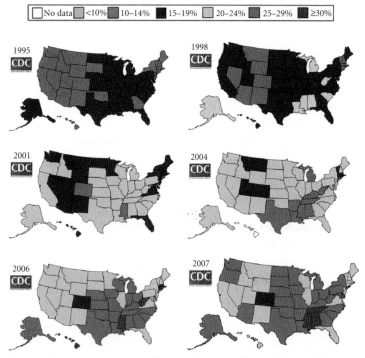

Fig. 2.4 Obesity trends among US adults from 1995 to 2007 (see also
Plate 1). Source: Centers for Disease Control (CDC) Behavioral Risk Factor
Surveillance System (BRFSS) 2007.

Factor Surveillance System, ten states had a prevalence of less than 10% in 1980 compared with no states with a prevalence that low in 1998. Whilst all states had a prevalence of less than 20% in 1995, only one state (Colorado) retained a prevalence of less than 20% by 2001. In 2007, the states with the greatest prevalence of obesity were Alabama, Mississippi, and Tennessee—all greater than 30%.

Childhood obesity Currently, 25% of the children in the USA are considered to be overweight and 11% are considered obese. Few gender difference exists among children in the USA in terms of the percentage who are overweight. Data from NHANES indicate an overall rise in the number of overweight US children between the ages of 2 and 19. Between 1971–1974 and 2003–2004, the number of overweight children increased in each age group: from 5 to 13.9% for children aged 2–5, from 4 to 18.8% for children aged 6–11, and from 6.1 to 17.4% for children aged 12–19.

Canada

Adult obesity According to the 2004 Canadian Community Health Survey (CCHS), 8.6 million or 36.1% of Canadian adults are overweight. An additional 5.5 million or 23.1% of Canadian adults are obese. Thus, a total of 59.2% of Canadian adults are over their healthy weight.

Although few gender differences exist in terms of the percentage of obese men and women (22.9 and 23.2%, respectively), a greater proportion of women than men are classified as class III obese. Figure 2.5 shows the breakdown of overweight and obese adults among the Canadian provinces by gender.

According to age group, 18–25-year-olds have the lowest prevalence of obesity with 10.7% for men and 12.1% for women. By contrast, 45–64-year-olds have the highest prevalence of obesity with approximately 30% for both men and women. Comparing the CCHS surveys for 1978–1979 and 2004, obesity rates have more than doubled among some age groups: from 9 to 21% for the age group 25–34, and from 11 to 24% for the age group 75+ years.

Childhood obesity Twenty-six percent of Canadian children are currently estimated to be overweight, with 500,000 or 8% of them obese. Few gender differences exist in terms of the percentage rise of

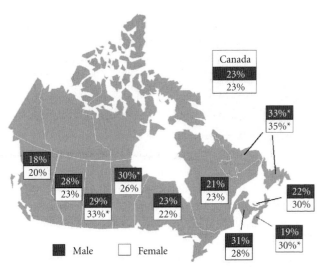

Fig. 2.5 Obesity rates among adults in Canada by province and gender. *indicates data significantly different from the overall estimate for Canada (P<0.05). Available at: http://www.statcan.gc.ca/pub/82-620-m/2005001/article/adults-adultes/8060-eng.htm. Source: CCHS 2.2 (2004), Statistics Canada.

overweight or obese children. For each sex, the combined percentage of children who are overweight and obese increased by 10% between 1978 and 2004 (from 17 to 27% for boys and from 15 to 25% for girls). According to age groups, trends differed between 1978 and 2004. For children aged 2–5, the prevalence of those at least overweight has remained at 21%, whilst the prevalence of obesity within that age range has risen from a negligible amount to 6%. For children aged 6–11, the proportion of children at least overweight has doubled from 13 to 26%, with the prevalence of obesity within those children increasing from a negligible amount to 8%. Finally, the proportion of children aged 12–17 who were at least overweight has doubled, and the proportion of obesity among children in the same age group has tripled.

Europe

Adult obesity Currently, in Europe, approximately 30% of adults are overweight and 10% of adults are obese. Figure 2.6 shows the current prevalence of obesity by gender among countries in Europe.

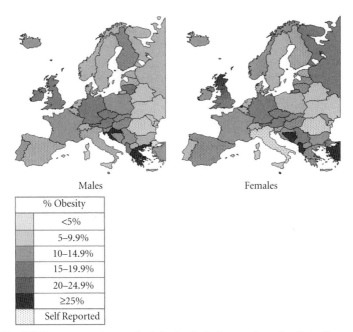

Males   Females

% Obesity
<5%
5–9.9%
10–14.9%
15–19.9%
20–24.9%
≥25%
Self Reported

Fig. 2.6 Current prevalence of adult obesity in Europe (see also Plate 2). Sources and references are available from obesity@iotf.org. © International Obesity TaskForce, London – October 2007.

The WHO estimates that obesity has risen by 10–40% in most European countries within the last 10 years. Figure 2.7 illustrates the rising trend in obesity within Europe during the past 20 years.

Childhood obesity Approximately 20% of children in Europe are overweight and one-third of those are obese. According to the IOTF, obesity among children in Europe has increased steadily. The highest prevalence of overweight children is found in southern Europe (20–35%), whilst Northern Europe has a prevalence of 10–20%.

Asia

According to WHO, the Asian countries with the highest prevalence of obesity include India, China, Indonesia, Japan, Pakistan, and Bangladesh. The IOTF estimates that obesity within Asia is increasing by about 1% a year, which is the same rate as Great Britain, the USA, and Australia.

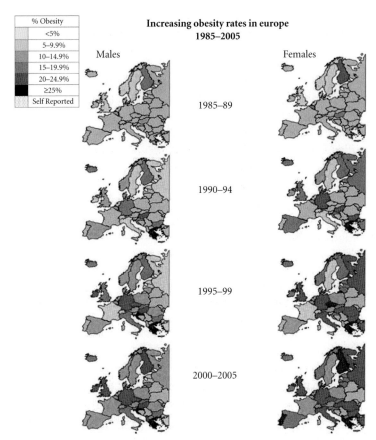

% Obesity
<5%
5–9.9%
10–14.9%
15–19.9%
20–24.9%
≥25%
Self Reported

Increasing obesity rates in europe
1985–2005

Males   Females

1985–89

1990–94

1995–99

2000–2005

Fig. 2.7 Rising trend of obesity in Europe from 1985 to 2005, by gender (see also Plate 3). With the limited data available, prevalences are not age standardized and data from different years are not always directly comparable. The illustrations above are to give an impression of the changes that have taken place over the last 20 years. Self-reported surveys (illustrated with dots) may underestimate true prevalence. Sources and references are available from obesity@iotf.org. © International Obesity TaskForce, London – October 2007.

Over 10% of children in many Asian countries are overweight, with rates of childhood obesity generally highest within urban areas.

China

A 2002 nutrition survey conducted within China indicated that, overall, 200 million people within China, or 22.8% of the population, were overweight, and 60 million, or 7.1%, were obese. Within Chinese cities, the percentage of overweight people has risen to 30%. Obesity within Chinese cities affects 12% of adults and 8% of children. In one rural province in China, a 2003–2004 survey revealed that 18.6% of the Chinese rural population were overweight (15.1% of men and 22.1% of women). Obesity affects 1.7% of the Chinese rural population, with 1.2% of men and 2.2% of women affected. Over 60 million Chinese people became obese between 1992 and 2002.

Indonesia

In Jakarta, Indonesia, a location at the cusp of its economic development, approximately 16% of pre-school-age children from high-income families were obese in 1995.

India

A study by the Nutrition Foundation of India found that middle-class groups had a higher prevalence of being obese and overweight than lower-income groups. In general, Indian females had a greater prevalence of being overweight/obese than males regardless of socioeconomic status or age. Whereas 32.2% of males and 50% of females were overweight among the middle-class groups, 1% of males and 4% females were overweight among lower-income groups. According to age, those over 40 years had the highest prevalence of obesity—3% of males and 14% of females.

Japan

Using the stricter BMI cut-off value for obesity of 25 kg/m^2, one in five adults in Japan is considered obese. For men over the age of 30 and women over the age of 40, the prevalence of obesity increases to 30%. Over the last 40 years, obesity among Japanese adults has increased three- to fourfold. According to the National Nutrition Survey, Japan, childhood obesity in Japan as of 2000 was 11.1% for boys and 10.2% for girls. Over the last 25 years, childhood obesity has increased by 6.1% for boys and 7.1% for girls.

Future trends

According to WHO's projections, 700 million adults worldwide are expected to be obese by 2015. WHO predicts that in the European region, approximately 150 million adults and 15 million children will be obese by 2010. The UK's Department of Health indicates that as many as 75% of men and 60% of women could be at least overweight by 2010. In the UK, 20% of British children are expected to be obese by 2010. The chairman of the IOTF predicts that, by 2010, 50% of children in North and South America are expected to at least be over-weight. In the European Union, the projected increase is up to 38% or 64 million. In China, one in five children is expected to be overweight. A 2007 study predicted that, in the USA, 75% of adults will be over-weight and 41% of adults will be obese by 2015. The prevalence of overweight children is expected to increase to 24% by the same year.

Key points

If current trends continue, various organizations and studies have predicted a steady rise in obesity in the future. In the European Union, the IOTF predicts that approximately 38% of children will be overweight by 2010. In North and South America, 50% of children are expected to be overweight by the same year. WHO predicts that obesity levels will increase worldwide to 700 million adults by 2015.

Chapter 3

Metabolically healthy obesity

Definition of metabolically healthy obesity

It is commonly assumed that obesity is associated with risks that predispose to cardiovascular disease. Although this concept remains generally true, recent and growing evidence shows that obesity is not necessarily associated with an unfavorable cardiometabolic profile.

In daily clinical practice, it is not unusual to see grossly obese subjects who do not have the traditional cluster of cardiometabolic risk factors. These obese individuals who are resistant to the development of adiposity-associated cardiometabolic abnormalities are defined as uncomplicated or metabolically healthy but obese (MHO) subjects. The existence of MHO subjects is not just a curiosity or a rarity, but a well-defined clinical entity.

These subjects are uncomplicated and do not express the common obesity-related clustering risk factors. MHO subjects present with lower waist circumference, normal lipid profile, normal blood pressure, normal glucose tolerance, and no signs or symptoms of coronary artery disease, despite large amounts of body fat. Morphological and functional cardiovascular risk markers are usually normal in MHO subjects or lower than you might expect from a person who is obese. In fact, these subjects have normal left ventricular mass, normal systolic function, normal or low carotid intima–media thickness (c-IMT) and normal liver enzymes. MHO subjects may also have lower inflammation and better insulin sensitivity than complicated obese subjects. However, these two aspects are relatively controversial and results are not univocal. The large variability in insulin sensitivity and the non-specific increased systemic inflammatory conditions that are commonly observed in obese subjects may be the reason for this controversy. The main characteristics of MHO subjects are summarized in Box 3.1.

Box 3.1 Features of MHO subjects

- Predominant subcutaneous peripheral adiposity
- Younger age when compared with complicated obese subjects
- Normal fasting glucose (≤100 mg/dl) and glucose tolerance (≤140 mg/dl during oral glucose tolerance test)
- Normal systolic and diastolic blood pressure values (≤120/80 mmHg)
- Normal lipid profile, including normal levels of triglycerides (≤150 mg/dl) and high-density-lipoprotein cholesterol (≥40 and ≥50 mg/dl in men and women, respectively)
- Lower prevalence of small low-density lipoprotein particles when compared with complicated obese subjects
- Better insulin sensitivity when compared with complicated obese subjects
- Lower inflammatory status when compared with complicated obese subjects
- Normal liver enzymes
- Normal resting electrocardiogram
- Appropriate echocardiographic left ventricular mass or no left ventricular hypertrophy
- Low c-IMT
- No clinical evidence of coronary artery disease or heart failure

Prevalence of metabolically healthy obesity

The prevalence of MHO subjects is unexpectedly high, with a wide range of 8–37% of obese subjects overall. Among US adults of 20 years and older, 31.7% of obese adults (approximately 19.5 million adults) are currently metabolically healthy. MHO subjects are equally likely to occur in all body mass index (BMI) categories, even when the BMI exceeds 50 kg/m^2. Uncomplicatedness seems to cross over both white European and North American populations. However, it is still unknown whether this obesity phenotype can be applied within all ethnic groups.

Correlates of metabolically healthy obesity

Although several possible convincing explanations have been proposed, the reasons for MHO subjects are not completely understood, and further clinical and research observations will be necessary. However, the best independent predictors of MHO subjects have been identified as a younger age and a smaller waist circumference. Hence, MHO subjects show a more prevalent subcutaneous, peripheral obesity phenotype rather than the central, visceral obesity phenotype typically observed in complicated morbidly obese subjects. MHO subjects can be considered a good explanatory model of how regional fat distribution is more important than overall obesity in predicting and stratifying the cardiovascular risk. Factors regulating lipid oxidation and lipogenesis in ectopic tissues such as the liver and muscle may be also relevant. Genetic variations in genes involved in lipid metabolism, such as adiponectin receptor-1 and hepatic lipase, as well as upstream transcription factor-1, displaying modulatory effects on hepatic lipase, may also represent candidate factors for a metabolically benign obesity. Higher physical activity levels and non-Hispanic black race/ethnicity have also been shown to correlate independently with the favorable cardiometabolic profile of MHO subjects. However, results regarding these two latter points are contradictory. Dietary, lifestyle, and environmental factors could also be considered as possible correlates of MHO.

Clinical management of metabolically healthy but obese subjects

MHO subjects also need clinical management and weight-loss strategies, similar to morbidly obese subjects. However, weight loss may be easier in MHO subjects than in complicated morbidly obese subjects. Their better insulin sensitivity and lower visceral adiposity may contribute to a better response to weight-loss interventions.

MHO subjects should be followed up prospectively in order to observe and possibly prevent the development of obesity-related complications.

These observations underline the need for better characterization and a re-definition of obesity in term of indices and classification. Anthropometric and imaging markers of regional fat distribution and insulin sensitivity indices may be more helpful in identifying morbidly obese and MHO subjects, independent of BMI.

Key points

MHO subjects are frequently observed in clinical practice. These subjects seem to have a protective obesity phenotype. MHO subjects are resistant to the development of traditional obesity-related clustering of cardiovascular factors. MHO subjects are generally younger and with more prevalent subcutaneous peripheral adiposity. They may also have better insulin sensitivity and lower inflammatory status. The reasons for this favorable cardiometabolic profile remain to be determined.

Chapter 4

Adipose tissue and the heart

Adipose tissue

A body of evidences clearly shows that the adipose tissue is not a silent fat 'storage room', but an active endocrine and paracrine organ serving as a source of several cytokines and hormones that can influence and modulate the cardiovascular system. Adipose tissue has been suggested to play an important role in the development of cardiovascular diseases. However, anatomical and biomolecular characteristics of human adipose tissue vary significantly. Because of their anatomical proximity to the internal organs, visceral fat depots are thought to play a major role in the development of morphological and functional changes in the heart and circulatory system. Increased adiposity can be accompanied by a number of metabolic and cardiovascular diseases that can independently affect the cardiovascular system. Hence, increased adiposity alone and its effect on the heart and cardiovascular system should be considered independently of other confounding factors.

Adipose tissue circulation

Adipose tissue is surrounded by an extensive capillary network. The fat cells, or adipocytes, are surrounded by stromal vascular cells, including endothelial cells. The adipocytes are located close to vessels with the highest permeability, the lowest hydrostatic pressure, and the shortest distance for transport of molecules to and from the adipocytes.

Adipose tissue compartments

Adipose tissue is not uniformly distributed throughout the human body, and its distribution is influenced by many factors, including sex, age, ethnicity, genotype, diet, physical activity level, and hormones. Human adipose tissue is not only located in different anatomic compartments, but also differs in terms of embryological origin and biomolecular properties, and hence differs in terms of therapeutic and diagnostic use.

In general terms, adipose tissue can be characterized as subcutaneous or visceral as shown in Figure 4.1. Subcutaneous adipose tissue and visceral adipose tissue are anatomically, biochemically, metabolically, and therefore clinically, different.

Subcutaneous adipose tissue

Subcutaneous adipose tissue is defined as the adipose tissue layer found between the dermis and the aponeuroses and fasciae of the muscles. Subcutaneous adipose tissue is generally distributed more in the peripheral regions of the human body, as well as the lower trunk, the gluteal thigh region, and around the abdominal circumference.

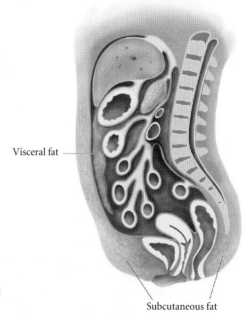

Visceral fat

Subcutaneous fat

Fig. 4.1 Visceral and subcutaneous abdominal adipose tissue.

Visceral adipose tissue

Visceral adipose tissue is the fat depot that surrounds the internal organs, including the heart, kidneys, and liver. There is a growing interest in analysis of different visceral adipose tissue subcompartments. Significant differences in the metabolic and functional properties of fat depots within visceral adipose tissue compartments have been suggested. Visceral adipose tissue is distributed among the three body cavities: intrathoracic, intra-abdominal, and intrapelvic. Intrathoracic adipose tissue includes epicardial, pericardial and mediastinal fat depots. Intra-abdominal adipose tissue also includes intraperitoneal adipose tissue as well as mesenteric and omental fat depots. This distribution is likely to require further subdivisions for each adipose tissue compartment in the body, based upon previously neglected and newly discovered human adipose tissue depots, as reported recently.

Due to its anatomic location and peculiar metabolic properties, as well as insulin resistance and pro-inflammatory, pro-thrombogenicity, and hyperlipolytic activity, an increased visceral adipose depot is a key correlate of the abnormal cardiometabolic risk profile observed in individuals with a visceral obesity phenotype. Increased portal release of free fatty acids, increased catecholamine-induced lipolysis, decreased activity of β_2-adrenoceptors, and decreased insulin-induced anti-lipolysis are characteristics of visceral fat depots. Regional variations in adipocyte lipolysis lead to more free fatty acids being released from visceral than from subcutaneous adipose tissue during hormone stimulation, as well as insulin and catecholamines. Differences in secretion of adipokines, such as resistin, leptin, adiponectin, plasminogen activator inhibitor-1 and angiotensinogen, between visceral and subcutaneous adipose depots may also contribute to a different cardiovascular and metabolic risk.

Abdominal visceral adipose tissue

Abdominal visceral adipose tissue can be defined as the visceral fat that is located within the abdominopelvic region. The abdominopelvic region includes intraperitoneal and extraperitoneal depots. The extraperitoneal component seems primarily to be a mechanical cushion for organs such as the kidneys, uterus, bladder, and large intestine, specifically the rectum. Metabolic, as well as anatomical, differences between intraperitoneal and retroperitoneal adipose tissue have been suggested. Intraperitoneal adipose tissue, which encompasses mesenteric and omental areas, is drained by the portal vein, whereas blood from retroperitoneal adipose tissue empties into the inferior vena cava. Intraperitoneal adipose tissue has been proposed to have a higher metabolic activity than retroperitoneal adipose tissue, independent of the size of the fat depot. The direct exposure of liver cells through the portal circulation to high concentrations of free fatty acids derived from intraperitoneal adipose tissue has been evoked to explain correlations between visceral adipose tissue and the metabolic syndrome components. Moreover, intraperitoneal fat depots have been proposed to account for the large proportion of inter-subject variation.

Increased visceral abdominal adiposity significantly impacts on the development of increased cardiovascular risk. Anthropometric markers of increased visceral abdominal adiposity are independently associated with increased risk of coronary artery disease among individuals with a body mass index (BMI) lower than 27 kg/m^2. Increased abdominal adiposity worsens the prognosis of patients with cardiovascular disease and increases the estimate of myocardial infarction attributable to obesity by threefold. Assessment of abdominal visceral fat is very important in the clinical management of obese subjects or individuals with increased visceral adiposity. Abdominal visceral fat can be measured indirectly by anthropometric surrogate markers or directly with more accurate imaging techniques.

Key point

Increased abdominal visceral fat is one of the key factors in obesity-associated cardiovascular diseases.

Epicardial adipose tissue

Epicardial and intra-abdominal fat evolve from brown adipose tissue during embryogenesis. In the adult human heart, epicardial fat is commonly found in the atrioventricular and interventricular grooves, extending to the apex. Minor foci of fat are also located subepicardially in the free walls of the atria and around the two appendages. As the amount of epicardial fat increases, it progressively fills the space between the ventricles, sometimes covering the entire epicardial surface. A small amount of adipose tissue also extends from the epicardial surface into the myocardium, often following the adventitia of the coronary artery branches. No muscle fascia divides epicardial fat and myocardium, and therefore the two tissues share the same microcirculation, as shown in Figure 4.2. As a result of the close anatomical relationship between epicardial adipose tissue and the adjacent myocardium, epicardial fat could locally modulate cardiac morphology and function in subjects with increased visceral adiposity.

Epicardial fat is metabolically very active. Epicardial adipose tissue has higher rates of fatty acid uptake and secretion than in other fat depots. Epicardial fat could therefore serve two distinct functions: (i) as a buffer, absorbing fatty acids and protecting the heart against high fatty acid levels, and (ii) as a possible local energy source at times of high demand, channeling fatty acids to the myocardium. Epicardial fat is also an important source of pro-inflammatory and pro-thrombotic

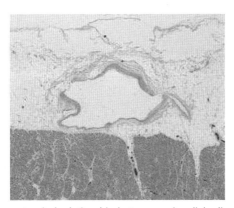

Fig. 4.2 Close anatomical relationship between epicardial adipose tissue and the adjacent myocardium, showing the absence of a muscle fascia between them (see Plate 4). Reproduced with permission from Iacobellis G, Corradi D & Sharma AM (2005) Epicardial adipose tissue: anatomical, biomolecular and clinical relation to the heart. *Nat Clin Pract Cardiovasc Med* 2:536–43.

adipokines and of the anti-inflammatory adiponectin. These products could affect the heart and coronary arteries through paracrine vasocrine mechanisms. Paracrine signaling can be defined as when adipokines secreted from epicardial adipocytes overlying the lipid core of atherosclerotic plaques diffuse into interstitial fluid across the adventitia, media, and intima, and interact respectively with the vasa vasora, vascular smooth muscle cells, endothelium, and the plaques. Vasocrine signaling can be defined as when adipokines secreted by epicardial adipocytes closely apposed to the adventitial vasa vasorum traverse the vessel into its lumen and are transported downstream to react with cells in the media and the intima around plaques.

Epicardial adipose tissue may also affect the left ventricular (LV) mass and LV diastolic function. Left, right, and total ventricular fat weights are significantly greater in hypertrophic hearts. Epicardial fat located over both ventricles accounts for around 20% of the total ventricular mass. By adding to the mass of the ventricles, increased epicardial fat increases the work of the heart in pumping blood. LV hypertrophy is associated with a consensual and proportional increase in epicardial fat mass, as depicted in Figure 4.3. In the hypertrophic heart, the adipose tissue also fills the epicardial spaces between the atrioventricular and interventricular grooves, and along the major

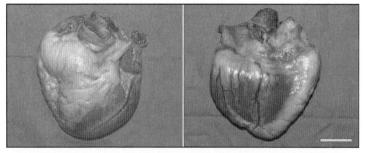

Fig. 4.3 Massive epicardial fat and eccentric cardiac hypertrophy. Bar, 4 cm. Reproduced with permission from Iacobellis G, Corradi D & Sharma AM (2005) Epicardial adipose tissue: anatomical, biomolecular and clinical relation to the heart. *Nat Clin Pract Cardiovasc Med* 2:536–43.

coronary branches. Increased epicardial fat mechanically affects LV diastolic filling and consequently induces atrial enlargement.

Key point

Epicardial fat may directly affect and modulate the heart and coronary arteries through mechanical, paracrine, and vasocrine mechanisms.

Mediastinal and pericardial adipose tissue

Recently, intrathoracic adipose tissue accumulation has also been evaluated. Ectopic fat deposition is not limited to the abdominal viscera, but may also occur in the thorax. Very few studies have previously focused their attention on this body fat compartment, which could be of great interest for evident anatomical reasons. Mediastinal and pericardial fat areas have been evaluated.

Mediastinal and pericardial adipose tissue are visceral fat depots that are accumulated intrathoracically and therefore exteriorly to the heart. A role for these fat depots has been suggested in adiposity-related cardiovascular diseases, but is still not completely understood. Increased mediastinal fat has been associated with increased blood pressure and insulin resistance. Pericardial fat is anterior to the epicardial fat and therefore located between visceral and parietal pericardium. Increased pericardial adipose tissue has been linked to coronary artery disease and atherosclerosis. Pericardial adipose tissue fat could also modulate coronary arteries.

Perivascular adipose tissue

Blood vessels are surrounded by varying amounts of perivascular adipose tissue. It is now clear that perivascular fat is not simply located around the arteries, but plays an active role in the regulation of vascular tone. Perivascular adipose tissue releases adipocyte-derived vascular relaxation factors. The modulation of vascular function by perivascular adipose tissue may be composed of a balance between relaxation and contraction factors. Alteration in perivascular fat properties may affect local sympathetic control of vascular tone.

Perivascular fat could potentially play a role in the morphological changes associated with an increase in vascular stiffness seen in obesity.

Intra-myocardial fat

Non-adipocytes as well as the cardiac cells have a very limited capacity to store excess fat. If they are exposed to high levels of plasma lipids, as usually occurs in obesity, they may undergo steatosis and loss of function, and ultimately cardiac lipotoxicity may occur. Cardiac lipotoxicity is associated with initial hypertrophy, followed by the development of LV dysfunction. Visceral adiposity induces fatty infiltration of the myocardium by different mechanisms. Two distinctly different patterns of myocardial fat deposition have been identified. The first pattern is characterized by an infiltration of adipocytes from the epicardial adipose tissue to areas between the myocardial fibers. The second pattern, formerly called 'fatty degeneration', is characterized by deposition of triacylglycerol droplets within the cytosol of the cardiomyocytes. In metabolic terms, the hypertrophied heart decreases its fatty acid use and increases its reliance on glucose as a fuel. The mechanisms involved in this substrate switching are complex. An overload of lipids in the myocardium induces ceramide production, which, through increased nitric oxide formation, can cause apoptosis of lipid-laden cells, such as cardiomyocytes. Ceramide accumulation may have a critical role in the pathogenesis of lipotoxic cardiomyopathy and lipoapoptosis in obesity. Excessive deposits of lipids within myocardial tissue could play an active role in the development of cardiovascular disease. Myocardial lipid content increases with the degree of adiposity and may contribute to the adverse structural and functional cardiac adaptations seen in obese subjects.

Effect of excess adiposity alone on myocardial metabolism

Abnormalities in myocardial metabolism may precede and contribute to cardiac dysfunction in obesity. Normally, the myocardium is able to utilize multiple substrates for metabolism, but in the post-natal state, it primarily uses fatty acids. In response to an increase in fatty acid delivery, the myocardium typically increases β-oxidation of fatty acids. If excessive fatty acid delivery to the myocardium persists, the myocardium's large capacity for fatty acid oxidation may be overwhelmed, causing increased fatty acid storage. Although much of this excess lipid may be stored in a relatively neutral form such as triglycerides, some of the fatty acids that enter the cell may contribute to apoptosis via lipotoxicity.

Epicardial adipose tissue has been suggested to play an active role in myocardial metabolism. The biochemical properties of epicardial adipose tissue have been studied in animal models and humans. In young adult guinea pigs, the rate of free fatty acid synthesis, release, and breakdown in response to catecholamines by the relatively small amount of epicardial adipose tissue was found to be markedly higher than in other adipose depots. The high lipolysis observed in epicardial adipose tissue could be due to several factors. The reduced anti-lipolytic effect of insulin in visceral adipose tissue and the increased activity of β-adrenergic receptors, especially $β_3$ receptors, could be suggested as possible mechanisms. Under physiological conditions, epicardial adipose tissue is thought to act as a buffering system against toxic levels of fatty acids between the myocardium and the local vascular bed. Thus, increased epicardial fat could scavenge excess fatty acids, which interfere with the generation and propagation of the contractile cycle of the heart, causing ventricular arrhythmias and alterations in repolarization. By contrast, the high lipolytic activity of epicardial fat suggests that this tissue might also serve as a ready source of free fatty acids to meet increased myocardial energy demands, especially under ischemic conditions. Obesity may also lead to mitochondrial alterations. Mitochondrial dysfunction and impaired myocardial metabolism may contribute to contractile dysfunction in the heart of obese individuals. Altered myocardial metabolism may differ with gender, age, and regional fat distribution. Increased interstitial fibrosis has also been described in the hearts of obese subjects. Fibrosis may ultimately lead to apoptotic cardiomyocyte death.

Effect of excess adiposity alone on cardiac morphology and function

Obesity is so closely related to its complications of hypertension, diabetes, glucose intolerance, dyslipidemia, and respiratory disease that it is difficult to distinguish the first pathological event that causes cardiac alterations.

Effect of excess adiposity alone on left ventricular geometry and systolic function

Isolated excess adiposity is actually related more to functional than to morphological modifications of the heart. Obese subjects exhibit increased muscle as well as adipose mass. Increased lean and fat mass and body surface area are associated with an increase in total blood volume, which contributes to an increase in LV preload and an increase in resting cardiac output. The increase in preload is also partially caused by hyperinsulinemia and its sodium-retentive action, although the lack of increased afterload and the low peripheral resistance that are commonly observed in normotensive obese subjects could also contribute.

The consequences of this adaptive mechanism are an increase in stroke volume, a supranormal systolic function, and possibly an enlargement in aortic root dimensions. The hyperdynamic systole seems to be necessary to supply higher oxygen consumption and energy demand due to an increase in body surface. However, in normotensive, non-diabetic, obese subjects, the hyperkinetic systole does not necessarily produce compensatory LV hypertrophy or pathological changes in LV geometry, but is associated with appropriate LV geometric changes and enlargement of the aortic root. Severe obesity (BMI >50 kg/m^2) in the absence of confounding and worsening co-morbidities is associated with adaptation and appropriate changes in cardiac structure and function, despite the massive amounts of fat tissue.

Thus, uncomplicated obese subjects may present an appropriate LV mass and good cardiac performance. Appropriateness of LV mass can be defined as when the increase in LV mass is higher than necessary to compensate for the increased workload. The degree of obesity does not seem to affect the appropriateness of LV mass and the systolic performance at rest.

An adaptive mechanism may occur in uncomplicated but severe obesity. However, uncomplicated but severe obesity may be also associated with a different LV remodeling, as shown in Figure 4.4.

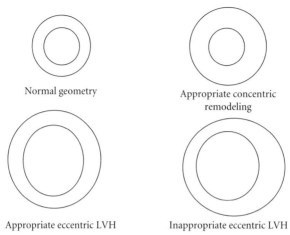

Normal geometry

Appropriate concentric remodeling

Appropriate eccentric LVH

Inappropriate eccentric LVH

Fig. 4.4 The most common left ventricle geometric patterns found in uncomplicated obesity.

Over time, the adaptation may become maladaptive and inappropriate LV geometric patterns can develop. Concentric LV remodeling, characterized by an increase in the relative wall thickness and normal LV mass, or eccentric LV hypertrophy can also be observed in normotensive obese subjects. Whether this maladaptive mechanism is a natural consequence of long-term obesity or is due to the occurrence of obesity-related co-morbidities is still unclear. Increased visceral adiposity is associated with higher LV mass and LV hypertrophy. In fact, subjects with central and abdominal fat accumulation frequently show abnormal LV geometry and mass. The effect of visceral fat on LV mass remains strong and independent of the traditional risk factors that can affect LV morphology. Increased cardiac adiposity, including both epicardial and pericardial fat depots, may also contribute to the development of inappropriate and maladaptive LV geometric patterns.

When hypertension and obesity occur together, it is likely that the increased pre-load may lead to inappropriate LV mass and a concentric and ultimately eccentric pattern of LV hypertrophy. Concentric LV hypertrophy can develop into eccentric hypertrophy with increased duration of obesity and the consequent increased duration of LV volume overload or as a long-term effect of hypertension. Obese patients with obstructive sleep apnea may develop right ventricle dilatation and hypertrophy due to the increased pulmonary blood pressure and insulin resistance.

Effect of excess adiposity alone on diastolic function

Obesity is commonly associated with diastolic dysfunction, independent of the co-existence of co-morbidities. The cause of diastolic dysfunction in obesity is not yet clear. It is likely that diastolic dysfunction in uncomplicated obesity could be caused by the combined effect of hemodynamic and metabolic factors. It has been suggested that LV diastole impairment can be altered by insulin resistance and hyperinsulinemia or by dysglycemia. Thus, insulin resistance may affect the biochemical mechanisms during diastolic relaxation by impairing the inactivation of myocardial actin–myosin cross-links attributable to a lack of Ca^{2+} re-uptake from the sarcoplasmic reticulum. Recent evidence indicates that excess visceral adiposity seems to be an independent cause of diastolic dysfunction. The cause–effect relationship of central obesity on diastole is independent of other traditional risk factors and is stronger than BMI. An increased epicardial fat pad has been also suggested to mechanically affect diastolic filling and relaxation.

Epicardial fat, a true visceral fat depot, may contribute directly towards impairing diastolic function in subjects with increased visceral adiposity.

Isolated excess adiposity is also associated with left atrial enlargement. This modification seems to be the consequence of diastolic dysfunction occurring in obesity. Increased left atrial size is a marker of chronic increased LV relaxation and filling pressures.

Adipokines and the cardiovascular system

It is now well known that the adipose tissue is not a silent 'storage room' for excess lipid, but is a metabolically active endocrine and paracrine organ, secreting a large number of proteins, hormones, growth factors, enzymes, and cytokines, known collectively as 'adipokines'.

The adipocyte, a mini-organ within this neglected organ, produces output signals (adipokines) and accepts input (via nuclear receptors). The adipose tissue communicates with almost all other organs through endocrine, paracrine, and also autocrine interactions. Both systemic and local regulation of the functions and morphology of internal organs have recently been attributed to the adipose tissue. Fat tissue is also a potential great responder, due to the presence of multiple receptors that can be modulated, stimulated, or inhibited by drugs with different mechanisms of action and therapeutic purposes.

Adipokines participate, both directly and indirectly, in the regulation of several processes that contribute to the development of hypertension, cardiac remodeling, inflammation, atherogenesis, thrombosis, and insulin resistance. Increased or abnormal fat mass can produce increased, decreased, or abnormal secretion of adipokines that can contribute to the development of obesity-associated cardiovascular diseases. The biochemical characteristics of the most important adipokines and their clinical implications in obesity are described briefly below.

Key points

Adipose tissue is an active endocrine and paracrine organ that secretes several adipokines that can directly or indirectly modulate the cardiovascular system. Increased adiposity is associated with increased, decreased, or abnormal production of adipokines with pro-inflammatory, pro-atherogenic, and pro-thrombotic or cardioprotective properties.

Adiponectin

Adiponectin is a protein mainly expressed by adipocytes. The local production of adiponectin by epicardial adipose tissue and cardiomyocytes suggests its autocrine–paracrine effect on the heart.

Adiponectin shows cardioprotective, anti-inflammatory, and anti-atherogenic properties. Adiponectin modulates myocardial remodeling after ischemic injury, attenuates cardiac hypertrophy and interstitial fibrosis, and protects against cardiomyocytes and capillary loss after myocardial infarction.

High plasma adiponectin concentrations are associated with a lower risk of acute coronary syndrome, myocardial infarction, and coronary heart disease.

Plasma adiponectin levels are reduced in patients with obesity, type 2 diabetes, and coronary artery disease. A low plasma adiponectin concentration is associated with impaired endothelial-dependent vasodilatation, concentric hypertrophy, and diastolic dysfunction.

Plasma adiponectin levels can be measured using commercial kits. Its use as a biochemical marker of cardiometabolic risk in clinical practice is currently under evaluation.

Leptin

Leptin is produced mainly by adipose tissue and participates in the control of body weight, the regulation of food intake, and energy expenditure. Leptin secretion is proportional to the amount of adipose tissue, and its plasma concentrations are markedly increased in obese individuals.

Leptin may play an important role in the pathogenesis of obesity-associated hypertension and LV hypertrophy. Leptin is also synthesized in cardiomyocytes and is released to the coronary effluent, suggesting that cardiac leptin may exert physiological effects on the myocardium.

Plasma leptin levels can be measured using commercial kits. Obese subjects show high leptin levels. The higher the BMI, the higher the leptin concentration. However, its value as a marker of cardiometabolic risk in obesity seems to be poor.

Resistin

Resistin is an adipokine expressed by macrophages and adipocytes. Resistin increases pro-inflammatory markers, upregulates the expression of adhesion molecules, promotes the release of endothelin-1 (ET-1) and stimulates the synthesis of monocyte chemoattractant protein-1 (MCP-1) in human endothelial cells. Resistin also induces endothelial dysfunction.

High plasma levels of resistin correlate with insulin resistance, pro-atherogenic inflammatory markers, unstable angina, congestive heart failure, and coronary atherosclerosis.

Serum resistin levels can be measured in obese subjects, but its clinical use remains unclear.

Ghrelin

Ghrelin is mainly produced by the stomach and intestine, but is also synthesized by the adipose tissue and cardiomyocytes. Ghrelin operates as an endogenous cardioprotective factor. It acts on the pituitary and hypothalamus to stimulate growth hormone release, food intake, and weight gain.

Ghrelin has cardiovascular effects through growth-hormone-dependent and -independent mechanisms. Intravenous administration of ghrelin in healthy individuals and patients with chronic heart failure improves cardiac function by increasing the cardiac index and the stroke volume index.

The potential of ghrelin in the treatment of severe cardiac heart failure is currently under investigation.

Angiotensinogen

The adipose tissue renin–angiotensin system produces angiotensinogen. Angiotensinogen produced in the adipose tissue and angiotensinogen-derived peptides, including angiotensin II, may influence adipogenesis and blood pressure. Increased angiotensinogen production by adipose tissue supports a role for the adipose renin–angiotensin system in hypertensive obese patients. Visceral adipose tissue expresses higher levels of angiotensinogen.

Plasminogen activator inhibitor-1

Plasminogen activator inhibitor-1 (PAI-1) is a major regulator of the fibrinolytic system, the natural defense against thrombosis. The major sources of PAI-1 synthesis are hepatocytes and endothelial cells, but adipocytes are also contributors.

The increased gene expression and secretion of PAI-1 by adipose tissue contribute to its elevated plasma levels in obesity. PAI-1 is correlated with fasting plasma insulin and triglycerides, BMI, and visceral fat accumulation.

Tumor necrosis factor-α

Tumor necrosis factor-α (TNF-α) is secreted by several adipose tissue depots. TNF-α is associated with obesity, inflammation, and insulin resistance. Weight loss in obese subjects may result in improved insulin sensitivity and a decrease in TNF-α levels. The plasma concentration of TNF-α can be measured, but its role in the pathogenesis of insulin resistance in obesity is still unclear.

Interleukin-6

Interleukin-6 (IL-6) is produced by human adipose tissue. Obese subjects may show higher circulating IL-6 levels than normoweight subjects. Increased IL-6 production by adipocytes may contribute to obesity-associated insulin resistance. IL-6 may modulate adipocytes through autocrine/paracrine mechanisms. Its clinical value is unknown.

Visfatin

Visfatin is a recently discovered adipokine that is produced mainly in visceral adipose tissue. The relationship between visfatin, obesity, and type 2 diabetes is controversial. The increase in visfatin synthesis associated with obesity and diabetes may represent a compensatory mechanism to maintain normoglycemia.

Adrenomedullin

Adrenomedullin is a potent vasodilator and anti-oxidative peptide. Adrenomedullin is produced by subcutaneous and visceral adipose tissue, including epicardial fat. Adrenomedullin may have a cardio-protective role.

Retinol-binding protein-4

Retinol-binding protein 4 (RBP4) is a protein secreted by adipocytes. RBP4 levels are elevated in the serum before the development of frank diabetes and it appears to identify insulin resistance and associated cardiovascular risk factors. However, circulating RBP4 concentrations seem to be similar in normoweight, overweight, and obese women.

C-reactive protein

C-reactive protein (CRP) is also secreted by adipocytes. CRP may be a marker of a chronic inflammatory state that can trigger acute coronary syndrome. Adiponectin and CRP expression in human adipose tissue appear to be linked.

Apelin

Apelin has been identified as the endogenous ligand of the orphan G protein-coupled receptor human APJ receptor. Apelin appears to provide cardioprotective effects and may be a promising target for the development of drugs to attenuate ischemic/reperfusion injury in patients with heart failure.

Osteopontin

Osteopontin is a phosphoprotein originally identified in osteoblasts and osteoclasts, but also secreted by adipocytes. Osteopontin may influence cardiovascular function, playing a role in atherosclerosis, LV hypertrophy, and cardiac fibrosis commonly associated with obesity. Circulating osteopontin levels are increased in obesity.

Endothelin-1

Endothelin-1 (ET-1) is a potent vasoconstrictor peptide. ET-1 is also produced by human adipocytes. Circulating ET-1 levels are increased in obese subjects. Circulating or adipose-derived ET-1 may promote systemic insulin resistance.

Nerve growth factor

Nerve growth factor (NGF) is a neurotrophic peptide also produced by human adipose tissue including epicardial fat. NGF is elevated in subjects with obesity and may contribute to coronary inflammation and atherosclerosis.

Chapter 5

Markers of adiposity

Anthropometric indices

Assessment of anthropometric indices is an essential part of obesity management in clinical practice. These indices are helpful in defining the degree of obesity, stratifying cardiometabolic risk, and reflecting regional fat distribution. Anthropometric indices should be part of a comprehensive health assessment of any individual with adiposity-related cardiovascular risk.

Anthropometric indices are non-invasive and unexpensive diagnostic and potentially prognostic tools in the management of obese patients. However, they are only surrogate markers of the degree of obesity and regional fat distribution, and therefore have several limitations; for example, they may provide incomplete information or be subject to operator variability. Imaging markers of adiposity are clearly superior in providing more accurate, reproducible, and reliable information.

The most commonly used anthropometric indices of obesity are:

+ Body mass index (BMI)
+ Waist circumference
+ Waist-to-hip ratio (WHR).

Key point

BMI and particularly waist circumference should be part of the routine clinical assessment of overweight and obese subjects and any individual with suspected increased regional adiposity.

Body mass index

Definition

Assessment of any patient should include an evaluation of BMI. BMI is a measure of body fatness based on height and weight that applies to both adult men and women.

Calculation

BMI is calculated as body weight in kilograms divided by height in meters squared (kg/m^2).

BMI cut-off points for overweight and obesity

Overweight and obesity are defined as a BMI $\geq$25 and $\geq$30 kg/m^2, respectively. Lower BMI thresholds appear to be more appropriate in Chinese and South-Asian populations.

Role of BMI in predicting cardiometabolic risk

Risk increases gradually as BMI increases from 25 to 29.9 kg/m^2 and rises more dramatically at a BMI of 30 kg/m^2, as shown in Table 5.1.

A higher BMI has traditionally been associated with a greater risk to health, with increasing BMI related to increasing risk of developing diabetes, glucose intolerance, hypertension, dyslipidemia, and coronary artery disease. Although this concept remains true, much clinical evidence has shown that the use of BMI may not be accurate in

Table 5.1 Cardiometabolic risk classification according to BMI

BMI category (kg/m^2)	Relative risk
Underweight (<18.5)	Increased risk
Normal weight (18.5–24.9)	Least risk
Overweight (25.0–29.9)	Increased risk
Obese	
Class I (30.0–34.9)	High risk
Class II (35.0–39.9)	Very high risk
Class III (≥40.0)	Extremely high risk

predicting cardiometabolic risk. The major criticism is based on the fact that BMI does not reflect regional fat distribution. In addition, BMI cannot discriminate between increased lean or fat mass. BMI can also be inadequate to classify the degree of obesity among different ethnic groups.

A higher BMI can provide a paradoxical protective effect and improves cardiovascular outcome in a subgroup of patients with congestive heart failure or who undergo cardiac surgery. This topic is addressed in Chapters 9 and 10. Moreover, a high BMI is not always associated with an unfavorable cardiometabolic profile, as has been learnt from metabolically healthy but obese subjects. These subjects present a high BMI (≥ 30 kg/m^2) but are free of major metabolic and cardiovascular obesity-related complications. This category of obese subject is discussed in detail in Chapter 3.

Despite this, measurement of BMI is simple, accurate, and helpful in population surveillance and in monitoring trends in the prevalence of obesity, and its use is still recommended in the clinical management of obese subjects.

Advantages of using BMI

◆ BMI provides a more accurate measure of total body fat than body weight alone

◆ BMI is a reliable indicator of total body fatness in both women and men

◆ BMI is a good marker of obesity-related cardiometabolic risk

◆ BMI correlates well with morbidity and mortality.

Limits of using BMI

◆ BMI is not an index of regional fat distribution

◆ BMI may overestimate body fat in athletes and individuals with a muscular build

◆ BMI may underestimate body fat in older persons and individuals who have lost muscle mass

◆ BMI may not reflect important ethnic differences in body composition.

Key points

BMI is an indicator of body fatness. The measurement of BMI is simple, accurate, and helpful in population surveillance and in monitoring trends in the prevalence of obesity. However, BMI cannot distinguish between individuals who have a similar build but significant differences in regional body fat distribution and fat content.

Waist circumference

Definition

Waist circumference provides an estimate of body girth at the level of the abdomen. Although specific techniques have been recommended for measuring waist circumference in the clinical setting, there is no uniformly accepted approach. The practical guidelines for a correct measurement of waist circumference in a clinical setting are shown in Figure 5.1.

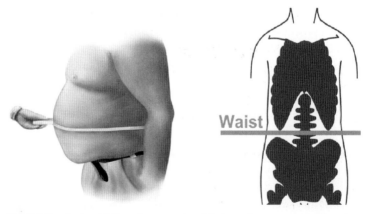

Fig. 5.1 Practical guidelines for correct waist circumference measurement. Place a tape measure around the bare abdomen, just above the hip bone. Be sure the tape is snug, but does not compress the skin. The tape should be parallel to the floor, midway between the top of the iliac crest and the lower rib margin on each side. The patient should relax and exhale while the measurement is made.

Role of waist circumference in predicting cardiometabolic risk

The importance of waist circumference in predicting cardiometabolic risk factors and adverse outcomes has been evaluated in many large epidemiological studies. A body of evidence shows that waist circumference is correlated with and predicts cardiovascular risk more powerfully than BMI. The role of waist circumference in predicting cardiovascular risk is independent and stronger than that traditionally attributed to BMI.

Waist circumference is considered an independent and powerful risk factor for coronary artery disease and myocardial infarction. Increased waist circumference is related to increased risk of diabetes, impaired glucose tolerance, hypertension, stroke, sleep apnea and dyslipidemia, independent of the degree of obesity. A large waist circumference is also an independent predictor of obesity-related cardiac abnormalities, as well as increased left ventricular mass, diastolic dysfunction, and excess epicardial fat. Increased waist circumference is also linked to inflammatory, atherogenic, and prothrombotic factors that are commonly overexpressed in subjects who are obese. Hence, the importance of waist circumference is directly related to the emerging importance of visceral adiposity as a cardiovascular risk factor, rather than overall obesity.

Waist circumference is a good surrogate index of visceral adiposity. Waist circumference correlates well with abdominal visceral fat measures obtained by imaging. In fact, waist circumference shows an excellent correlation with both magnetic resonance imaging (MRI) and computed tomography (CT) imaging of intra-abdominal visceral fat accumulation. Waist circumference is also correlated with CT-detected coronary calcium content and echocardiographic epicardial fat thickness. Intuitively, waist circumference measurement is cheaper and easier than imaging procedures, although imaging provides more precise and accurate information.

The recommended waist circumference thresholds for increased cardiometabolic risk in both men and women are reported in Table 5.2. Values of ≥88 cm in women and ≥102 cm in men indicate substantially increased risk.

Table 5.2 Waist circumference thresholds for increased cardiometabolic risk

	Increased risk	Substantially increased risk
Men	≥94 cm	≥102 cm
Women	≥80 cm	≥88 cm

Table 5.3 Cardiometabolic risk relative to BMI and waist circumference

Class	BMI (kg/m²)	Men ≤102 cm Women ≤88 cm	Men ≥102 cm Women ≥88 cm
Underweight	18.5	–	–
Normal	18.5–24.9	–	–
Overweight	25.0–29.9	Increased	High
Obesity (class I)	30.0–34.9	High	Very high
Obesity (class II)	35.0–39.9	Very high	Very high
Extreme obesity (class III)	≥40	Extremely high	Extremely high

Waist circumference can identify overweight subjects who are at increased cardiovascular risk but who would not otherwise be identified by fitting into normal or overweight categories. The World Health Organization (WHO) Obesity Task Force has proposed a classification system based on waist circumference as shown in Table 5.3. In addition, given the fact that cardiovascular risk varies significantly with ethnicity, waist circumference is a helpful index of visceral adiposity among different racial groups. However, because of the significant differences in body size among different ethnic groups, specific high-risk waist circumference values have been proposed for each ethnic group, as summarized in Table 5.4.

Advantages of using waist circumference

- Waist circumference correlates with abdominal visceral fat
- Waist circumference is considered a reliable marker of visceral adiposity

Table 5.4 Ethnic-specific values for waist circumference

Country or ethnic group	Men	Women
European	≥94 cm	≥80 cm
South Asian, Chinese	≥90 cm	≥80 cm
Japanese	≥85 cm	≥90 cm
South and Central American	Use South Asian cut-off points until more specific data is available	
Sub-Saharan African	Use European cut-off points until more specific data is available	
Eastern Mediterranean and Middle East (Arab)	Use European cut-off points until more specific data is available	

- Waist circumference is an important predictor of diabetes, coronary artery disease, and mortality rate, independent of BMI, blood pressure, blood glucose, and lipid profile

- Waist circumference provides an incremental value in predicting diabetes, coronary heart disease, and mortality rate compared with that provided by BMI

- Waist circumference can identify overweight subjects who are at increased cardiovascular risk but who would not otherwise be identified by having a BMI ≥25 kg/m^2

- In some ethnic groups, such as Chinese and South-Asians, waist circumference is a better indicator of relative disease risk than BMI

- Waist circumference is a better risk estimate for obesity-related disease in elderly subjects than BMI

- Monitoring changes in waist circumference may provide an estimate of abdominal fat changes, even in the absence of a change in BMI.

Limits of using waist circumference

- Waist circumference is not an accurate marker of visceral adiposity

- Waist circumference may not be an accurate indicator of abdominal visceral fat in severely obese subjects (BMI ≥40 kg/m^2)

- Waist circumference measurement requires specific training to ensure that reliable data are obtained

- ◆ Waist circumference measurement is subject to intra-operator and inter-operator variability
- ◆ Ethnic and age-related differences in body fat distribution may modify the predictive validity of waist circumference as a surrogate marker of abdominal fat.

Key points

Waist circumference is a surrogate marker of visceral adiposity. Waist circumference predicts adiposity-related cardiometabolic risk independently and better than BMI. A waist circumference ≥88 cm in women and ≥102 cm in men indicates substantially increased risk. Waist circumference is a helpful tool in the clinical management of subjects with increased visceral fat and increased cardiovascular risk who do not necessarily fit into the obese categories as defined by BMI. Measuring waist circumference requires expertise and accuracy. It may be subject to operator variability and may lose sensitivity in severely obese subjects.

Waist-to-hip ratio

Definition

Waist-to-hip ratio (WHR) is calculated as waist circumference divided by hip circumference. WHR is a marker of visceral fatness.

Measurement

Waist circumference is measured as described above. The hip measurement is taken at the widest level over the trochanters. Waist and hip measurements are taken twice, and the means of the measurements are used to calculate WHR.

Role of waist-to-hip ratio in predicting cardiometabolic risk

A WHR of ≥0.95 or ≥0.8 indicates increased cardiovascular risk in men and women, respectively.

WHR is a powerful independent predictor of hypertension, diabetes mellitus, and coronary artery disease.

Waist circumference and WHR are widely used as indicators of abdominal obesity. Whether WHR is superior to waist circumference in reflecting visceral adiposity and predicting cardiovascular risk is controversial and the subject of debate. The majority of current studies show that waist circumference is probably a better indicator of visceral fat and is more strongly correlated with cardiovascular risk factors than WHR, whereas others demonstrate that WHR has the strongest association with cardiovascular diseases.

The inclusion of hip circumference within the WHR may explain some of these differences. Hip circumference reflects femoral and gluteal subcutaneous fat. Hip circumference in women can be explained mostly by variations in gluteal fat mass and pelvic width, whereas in men, muscle mass can be the main determinant of hip circumference.

Whether hip circumference has an independent correlation with cardiometabolic risk and whether this association is positive or negative remains unclear.

Key points

WHR is a marker of visceral fatness. A WHR of ≥ 0.95 or ≥ 0.8 indicates increased cardiovascular risk in men and women, respectively. Whether WHR is superior to waist circumference in reflecting visceral adiposity and predicting cardiovascular risk is controversial.

Imaging of adiposity

Regional fat distribution and imaging

Visceral and subcutaneous are the major adipose tissue compartments in the human body. They are anatomically, biochemically, and clinically different. Studies have clearly shown that regional body fat distribution plays a major role in differentiating cardiometabolic risk. Visceral fat, that is the fat depot close to the internal organs, is considered to be one of the main factors in obesity-related cardiovascular abnormalities, as mentioned earlier. In particular, increased abdominal, cardiac, and upper-trunk visceral fat depots have been reported to be correlated with an unfavorable cardiometabolic profile.

Quantification of adipose tissue compartments, especially the visceral fat depot, is therefore very important for cardiovascular risk stratification and prediction in subjects with increased adiposity and obesity. Changes in regional fat distribution can be also targeted during therapeutic interventions and weight-loss strategies.

Imaging techniques are the most precise and reliable methods for qualitative and quantitative adipose tissue calculation. Several imaging methods have been proposed for estimation of both visceral and subcutaneous adiposity. Magnetic resonance imaging (MRI) and computed tomography (CT) are considered the reference methods for adipose tissue quantification. Main visceral fat depots can be detected and measured by MRI and CT. Comparison between MRI and CT shows a high degree of agreement in adipose tissue measurement, although the coefficient of variation for visceral adipose tissue measurements by CT is lower than that observed by MRI. Multi-detector computed tomography (MDCT) has emerged as a new and accurate technique for quantitative measurements of adipose tissue compartments. Ultrasound methodologies can provide cost-effective, non-invasive, accurate, and reliable quantification of some visceral adipose tissue compartments, whilst proton magnetic resonance spectroscopy (^{1}H-MRS) is a non-invasive method for measurement of intracellular lipid content.

Imaging of visceral fat

There is a growing interest in analysis and measurement of different visceral adipose tissue subcompartments. Significant differences in the metabolic and functional properties of depots within visceral adipose tissue compartments have been suggested. Visceral adipose tissue consists of adipose tissue that is distributed mainly in the three body cavities: intrathoracic, intra-abdominal, and intrapelvic adipose tissue. However, most studies have defined visceral fat as intra-abdominal only, with a range from 5 cm below L4–L5 to the slice corresponding to the superior border of the liver. This is the most frequently measured compartment. Some reports have included the sum of intra-abdominal and intrapelvic fatty tissues for visceral fat calculation. Visceral fat measurements range anatomically from the femoral heads to the liver dome or base of the lungs. MRI imaging of this area has been measured within the seven slices of 10 mm with 40 mm spaces between slices extending from two below and four above the L4–L5 level. This area could be defined as the abdominopelvic region, and prior observations support the hypothesis that sections taken from above L4–L5 contain more metabolically active visceral fat. In addition, visceral fat areas 5–10 cm above L4–L5 have been shown to have better correlations with visceral adipose tissue than areas at the traditional L4–L5 location.

Multi-slice volume and whole-body imaging are considered to be the references for measuring total and regional adipose tissue volumes. Circular, and more recently elliptical, models are used to estimate the cross-sectional abdominal visceral fat area. However, the relatively high cost of whole-body scans using MRI and the exposure to radiation of CT have led to the use of single-slice studies for this application. Single-slice imaging has had controversial results. The accuracy of a single cross-sectional image area in estimating or representing visceral adipose tissue volume is not well established. Some studies have reported a good correlation between visceral fat area measured in a single slice and visceral adipose tissue volume measured by using multiple slices whereas others have not. Although single-slice MRI appears to be a good tool in interventional and large studies, multiple-slice MRI imaging provides a more accurate visceral fat measurement. However, single-slice studies can evaluate smaller adipose tissue compartments and enhance metabolic differences among visceral adipose tissue depots.

Comparison of magnetic resonance imaging and computed tomography in measuring adipose tissue

MRI and CT are both considered to be gold standard techniques for total and visceral adipose tissue measurement. Both procedures are accurate and highly reproducible and there is no substantial superiority of one technique over the other one. However, some advantages can be identified for each.

CT is an excellent tool for assessment of human body fat compartments. CT provides high reproducibility in calculating adipose tissue volume. The subcompartments of adipose tissue, that is visceral and subcutaneous adipose tissue, can be measured accurately with minimal errors of 1.2 and 0.5%, respectively. CT can be easier to use than MRI. However, CT involves ionizing radiation. Radiation exposure makes it unsuitable for multiple-image whole-body tissue quantification and for use in children and pre-menopausal women. Some inaccuracy can be caused by bone tissue, which scatters radiation.

MRI is an excellent method for measuring adipose tissue compartments. In contrast to CT, MRI does not use radiation. MRI can also be used to assess lipid infiltration in tissues such as muscle and the liver. However, although MRI measurements of subcutaneous fat are almost identical to those obtained with CT, visceral adipose tissue may be slightly underestimated by MRI. MRI has advantages over CT in fat measurements of bony areas such as thighs and hips. MRI estimation of adipose tissue compartments can be an expensive, time-consuming, and labor-intensive process. MRI measurements can take a longer time to complete and movement artifacts can be a problem In addition, MRI availability and routine use may be limited.

Limitations of MRI in obese patients

MRI image quality is less affected by obesity than CT scans, although increased physique introduces noise and the large field of view required decreases the in-plane resolution of the images. Obesity can affect MRI scanning times. The main limitations for MRI are the size of the bore and the table weight limits, which may prevent imaging of large patients. MRI bore diameters (maximum aperture diameter is 60 cm for cylindrical-bore MRI and 55 cm for vertical-field MRI) are smaller than those of CT scanners and contact with the bore creates eddy currents that degrade magnetic resonance images.

Vertical-field MRI has a higher weight capability (up to 250 kg), but is not always available. It can be used to image larger patients, but generally offers lower field strength, resulting in degraded image quality and longer examination times, causing patient discomfort and motion artifact on images. It cannot be used to perform examinations requiring dynamic intravenous contrast administration.

Limitations of CT in obese patients

The patient's weight and girth can be a serious practical limit in CT imaging. The weight limit for CT tables is usually 200 kg, depending on the scanner. The bore of the gantry has a diameter of 70 cm, which is sometimes too small for patients who do not exceed the weight limit. Increases in gantry diameter on the newer, larger-gantry CT scanners permit increases in the field of view to accommodate larger patients.

Magnetic resonance imaging of adipose tissue

MRI is considered the reference technique for the measurement of both visceral and subcutaneous adipose tissue (Figure 5.2). MRI is able to quantify adipose tissue volume as voxels or volume elements. MRI visceral fat measurements are reported as either area values (cm^2) obtained from a single image, or as volume values (cm^3) derived using the tissue area measurements from multiple images and inserting these values into a mathematical algorithm. The calculation of adipose tissue area on a given MRI image is performed by subjecting the data to various segmentation techniques and determining the area by multiplying the number of pixels in the highlighted region by their known area.

Specific computer software programs for MRI analysis of adipose tissue have been developed. In one of the most commonly used, the

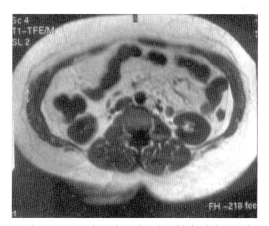

Fig. 5.2 Magnetic resonance imaging showing high abdominal visceral and subcutaneous fat depots (white signal) in an obese patient. Image from the author's collection.

volume of a tissue for the whole body or a given region to be analyzed is derived in two steps. Firstly, the volume for each image is derived by multiplying the area of the tissue by the slice thickness. The whole-body or regional volume is then calculated using a mathematical algorithm. A three-dimensional formula derives the volume of a given tissue by adding the volumes of truncated cones defined by pairs of consecutive images. A two-dimensional circular model is typically used to estimate cross-sections of abdominal visceral fat area. This model is based on two assumptions: (i) the cross-section of a human abdomen is a circle, and (ii) the visceral compartment (peritoneal cavity and its muscle wall) and the surrounding subcutaneous adipose tissue layer constitute two concentric circular areas. However, it has recently been noted that the cross-sectional shapes of a typical abdomen and, in particular the visceral compartment, are in fact closer to ellipses than circles, and therefore an elliptical model to estimate visceral adipose tissue has been developed. Measurement of visceral adipose tissue is now performed using the elliptical model, which has a stronger association with MRI-determined visceral adipose tissue than the circular model. A phantom (a complex plastic simulation of a human torso) to simulate the distribution of subcutaneous and intra-abdominal fat has also been created. Axial MRI images are obtained twice through the phantom using a 5 mm slice thickness and zero gap for the following T1-weighted sequences: spin echo, fast Dixon, and three-dimensional spoiled gradient echo. The T1-weighted three-dimensional spoiled gradient echo sequence generated similar ratios of intra-abdominal to subcutaneous adipose tissue in a fraction of the acquisition time. A methodology that allows the automatic processing of MRI axial images, segmenting the adipose tissue by a fuzzy clustering approach, has been also proposed. The use of an active contour algorithm on image masks provided by the fuzzy clustering algorithm allows the separation of subcutaneous fat from visceral fat. Visceral adipose tissue is calculated by an automated procedure based on automatic image histogram analysis.

Abdominal fat

Objective and accurate assessment of visceral fat is key in stratifying cardiometabolic risk in subjects with increased adiposity. An increased

MRI visceral fat area is associated with higher cardiometabolic risk in overweight and obese subjects. Prospective studies have shown that intra-abdominal fat predicts future hypertension and type 2 diabetes, independent of age, BMI, and weekly energy expenditure.

MRI of abdominal visceral adipose tissue is measured at the L4–L5 level, which corresponds to the superior border of the liver. A visceral fat area ≥ 130 cm^2 is generally used as the cut-off point to indicate high intra-abdominal adiposity. A visceral fat area ≥ 110 cm^2 has also been proposed to define high intra-abdominal visceral adiposity in obese women.

Epicardial fat

MRI can be used to quantify epicardial adipose tissue, the visceral fat depot surrounding the heart. Epicardial fat MRI scans can be obtained by a turbo spin echo with T1-weighting sequences with oblique axial orientation for a correct study of the four cardiac chambers.

Two individuals may present with the same BMI but very different epicardial fat and metabolic profiles, as shown in Figure 5.3.

Intrathoracic and pericardial fat

MRI can be used to measure mediastinal and pericardial fat depots, which are markers of intrathoracic adiposity (Figure 5.4). Increased intrathoracic adiposity is associated with hypertension and metabolic syndrome.

Ectopic fat

Although magnetic resonance spectroscopy (^{1}H-MRS) is considered the gold standard imaging technique, MRI can also be used to assess ectopic fat deposition within the muscle and liver. The Dixon method is most commonly used to measure fatty infiltration by MRI. Basically, fat and water proton content produces different signals. This implies that fat signal intensity of a given region relative to its water signal intensity can be used as a marker of lipid infiltration. However, with this methodology, MRI cannot separate the lipid into its intra- and extracellular lipid compartments. This may be important, as lipid accumulation can have different metabolic consequences depending on whether it is inside or outside the muscle cells.

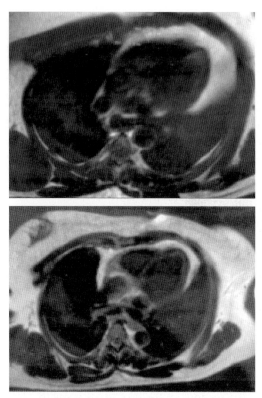

Fig. 5.3 Magnetic resonance imaging of epicardial fat in subject with complicated severe visceral obesity (top image) and in a subject with predominant peripheral obesity and no metabolic complications (bottom image). Epicardial fat mass is significantly higher in the subject with visceral adiposity. Reproduced with permission from Iacobellis G, Leonetti F & Di Mario U (2003) Massive epicardial adipose tissue indicating severe visceral obesity. *Clin Cardiol* 26:237, with permission of John Wiley & Sons, Inc.

Computed tomography imaging of adipose tissue

In addition to MRI, CT is also considered the reference standard for evaluation of adipose tissue. Briefly, CT uses ionizing radiation and differences in tissue X-ray attenuation to produce cross-sectional images of the body. X-ray attenuation is commonly expressed in Hounsfield units (HU). Low-density tissues such as adipose tissue have lower HU ratings than high-density tissues such as muscle

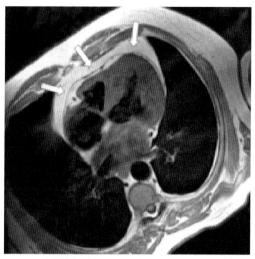

Fig. 5.4 Magnetic resonance imaging (MRI) of mediastinal fat. Arrows indicate the pericardium separating intrapericardial and extrapericardial adipose tissue. The MRI scan was obtained by fast-spin echo T1-weighted sequences. Reproduced with permission from Sironi A M, Gastaldelli A & Mari A (2004) Visceral fat in hypertension: influence on insulin resistance and β-cell function. *Hypertension* 44:127.

or bone. Cross-sectional CT images are composed of many pixels, each with an HU value reflecting the molecular composition of the tissue. CT images are normally analyzed using one of two methods: (i) the perimeter of the tissue is traced manually and the area within the perimeter is calculated by multiplying the number of pixels in the region of interest by their known area, or (ii) image segmentation algorithms are used to identify all pixels within a selected range of intensities (i.e. HU). The latter method is the most commonly used. Because of the radiation involved with CT, multiple CT images are generally not acquired. However, if multiple images are acquired, tissue volumes are calculated with the same methods used for MRI. They can then be converted to mass units by multiplying the volume by the assumed density values for that tissue.

CT imaging of abdominal fat

CT imaging of visceral intra-abdominal and subcutaneous abdominal areas is measured at the level of L4–L5, as for MRI. In obese subjects, the CT scan area should also be defined in relation to the skeleton and body phenotype.

In obese subjects, the level of the umbilicus, which has been proposed as an alternative anatomical landmark, can change from one patient to another, thus changing the visceral adipose tissue area. Hence, it may be advisable not to use the umbilicus as a landmark in these subjects.

As with MRI, an increased CT visceral fat area is associated with unfavorable cardiometabolic risk in overweight and obese subjects.

Multi-detector computed tomography

Multi-detector computed tomography (MDCT) is an emerging technique used to quantify the adipose tissue compartments. MDCT-based volumetric quantification of abdominal adipose tissue is highly reproducible. Volumetric measurements can depict age- and gender-related differences of visceral and subcutaneous abdominal adipose tissue deposition.

MDCT imaging of epicardial fat   Epicardial fat thickness and volume surrounding the coronary arteries can be quantified by MDCT (Figure 5.5). At each of the three main coronary territories, maximal

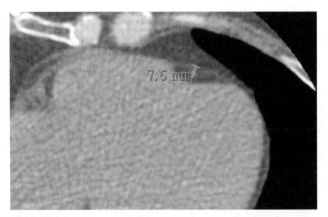

Fig. 5.5 Multi-detector computed tomography scan showing the pericardium with the epicardial adipose tissue beneath it surrounding the left anterior descending coronary artery. Adapted with permission from de Vos AM, Prokop M, Roos CJ, et al. (2008) Peri-coronary epicardial adipose tissue is related to cardiovascular risk factors and coronary artery calcification in post-menopausal women. *Eur Heart J* 29:777–83.

epicardial fat thickness (measured in mm) is determined perpendicular to the pericardium. Levels of MDCT-determined epicardial fat are related to coronary artery disease and coronary calcium levels. The coronary calcium score is significantly higher in patients with increased epicardial fat volume. In addition, in women, higher peri-coronary epicardial adipose tissue thickness is related to increased age, higher BMI, systolic blood pressure, triglycerides and glucose levels, larger waist circumference and WHR, and lower high-density lipoprotein levels than women with a lower peri-coronary epicardial adipose tissue thickness.

Key points

MRI and CT are considered the reference techniques for the measurement of adipose tissue. MRI and CT are used to calculate abdominal visceral adipose tissue at the L4–L5 level, which corresponds to the superior border of the liver. A visceral fat area ≥ 130 cm^2 is generally used as the cut-off point to indicate high intra-abdominal adiposity. MRI and CT can be also used to quantify epicardial, pericardial, and mediastinal adipose tissue. CT can be more accurate in measuring visceral fat, but MRI provides results substantially similar to CT without exposure to ionizing radiation.

Ultrasound imaging of visceral adipose tissue

Quantification of visceral fat is a helpful and practical diagnostic tool for the clinician committed to managing obese patients with cardiovascular disease or with high cardiovascular risk. Ultrasound can be an effective tool for practical and easy assessment of visceral body fat.

Advantages of ultrasound in assessing fat

Ultrasound can be used in clinical practice for the routine assessment of regional adiposity. Ultrasound is non-invasive, cost-effective, and accessible, and ultrasound techniques are simple and reproducible. Ultrasound assessment of visceral adiposity is a good alternative to the more sophisticated and expensive techniques described above.

Limitations of ultrasound in assessing fat

Ultrasound images, particularly abdominal ultrasound images, can be affected by large amounts of fat. Ultrasound energy is attenuated by fat tissue, especially at higher frequencies.

Ultrasound provides a linear measurement than cannot reflect the total volume of the fat tissue depot. Ultrasound may also be less accurate than MRI, CT, and MDCT imaging techniques. However, among the ultrasound techniques that have been developed in recent years, echocardiographic quantification of epicardial fat thickness seems to provide accurate and reproducible information on visceral adiposity.

Solutions to improving image quality in obese patients include using the lowest frequency transducer available (2 MHz), positioning the transducer to image the organ of interest within the range of the focal length of the transducer, and examining the patient's previous images to determine the thickness of subcutaneous fat.

Echocardiographic measurement of epicardial fat thickness Epicardial fat can be measured with two-dimensional standard echocardiography. Clinical assessment of echocardiographic epicardial fat is rapidly growing as a diagnostic tool for cardiometabolic risk stratification.

Echocardiographically, epicardial fat is identified as the echo-free space between the outer wall of the myocardium and the visceral layer of pericardium, and its thickness is measured perpendicularly on the free wall of the right ventricle (RV) at end systole in three cardiac cycles (Figure 5.6a). Because it is compressed during diastole, maximum epicardial fat thickness is measured in end systole. Epicardial fat is also identified as hyperechoic space, if it is present in large amounts (>15 mm) (Figure 5.6b). Parasternal long- and short-axis views permit the most accurate measurement of epicardial adipose tissue on the RV, with optimal cursor beam orientation in each view. Maximum epicardial fat thickness is measured at the point on the free wall of the RV along the midline of the ultrasound beam, perpendicular to the aortic annulus, used as an anatomical landmark for this view. For mid-ventricular parasternal short-axis assessment, maximum epicardial fat thickness is measured on the RV free wall along the midline of the ultrasound beam, perpendicular to the interventricular septum at

(a)

(b)

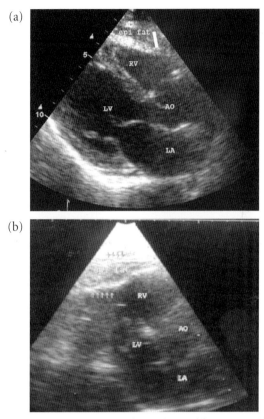

Fig. 5.6 Echocardiographic epicardial fat thickness. (a) Parasternal long-axis view showing epicardial fat (epi fat) as the echo-free space between the outer wall of the myocardium and the visceral layer of the pericardium. (b) Modified parasternal long-axis view showing large (>15 mm) epicardial fat hyperechoic space between the outer wall of the myocardium and the visceral layer of pericardium. LV, left ventricle; RV, right ventricle; LA, left atrium, AO, aorta. Reproduced with permission from Iacobellis G, Willens HJ, Barbaro G & Sharma AM (2008) Threshold values of high-risk echocardiographic epicardial fat thickness. *Obesity* 16:887–92.

the mid-chordal and tip of the papillary muscle level as the anatomical landmark. The mean value of three cardiac cycles from each echocardiographic view is used.

Epicardial fat needs to be distinguished from pericardial fat. Pericardial fat can be identified as the hypoechoic space anterior to the epicardial fat and parietal pericardium, and does not change size significantly during the cardiac cycle.

Inter- and intra-observer agreement on epicardial fat thickness measurement is excellent: the inter- and intra-class coefficients of correlation are 0.90 and 0.98, respectively.

The echocardiographic epicardial fat thickness range varies from a minimum of 1 mm to a maximum observed value of 25 mm. Echocardiographic epicardial fat is associated with MRI of visceral abdominal fat and waist circumference. Given the high cost of MRI and poor sensitivity of waist circumference, this ultrasound technique can easily be applied in clinical practice for visceral fat assessment. Echocardiographic epicardial fat is correlated with indices of insulin resistance and glucose tolerance, and with carotid intima–media thickness (c-IMT), an index for subclinical atherosclerosis. Echocardiographic epicardial fat is also a sensitive marker of changes in visceral fat associated with weight loss and is therefore a useful therapeutic target. Echocardiographic epicardial fat thickness cut-off values of 9.5 mm in men and 7.5 mm in women are predictive of metabolic syndrome and high intra-abdominal fat, as shown in Table 5.5.

Advantages of echocardiographic imaging of epicardial fat As echocardiography is performed routinely in high-risk overweight/obese patients, this objective non-invasive measure may be available at no extra cost. Echocardiographic assessment of epicardial visceral fat is certainly less expensive than MRI and CT. Echocardiographic measurement of epicardial fat thickness is simple and reproducible, and for measurement of visceral adipose tissue it provides a more sensitive and specific measure of true visceral fat content, avoiding the possible confounding effect of increased subcutaneous abdominal fat. Echocardiographic epicardial fat may be a more reliable quantitative therapeutic target during interventions to modulate and reduce

Table 5.5 Predictive values of epicardial fat thickness for metabolic syndrome and abdominal fat

	Men	Women
Metabolic syndrome*	≥9.5 mm	≥7.5 mm
High abdominal fat[†]	≥9.5 mm	≥7.5 mm
Extremely high abdominal fat[‡]	≥13 mm	≥10 mm
Insulin resistance[§]	≥9.5 mm	≥9.5 mm
High insulin resistance[||]	≥11 mm	≥11 mm

*As defined by Adult Treatment Panel III criteria.

†Defined as waist circumference >102 cm and >88 cm in men and women, respectively.

‡Defined as waist circumference >120 cm and >100 cm in men and women, respectively.

§Defined as a HOMA-IR (homeostasis model assessment of insulin resistance) value of 2.7–7.

||Defined as a HOMA-IR value of ≥7.

Adapted with permission from Iacobellis G, Willens HJ, Barbaro G & Sharma AM (2008) Threshold values of high-risk echocardiographic epicardial fat thickness. *Obesity* 16:887–92.

visceral adiposity. Retrospective analysis of echocardiograms and imaging can be obtained, even if they were not specifically performed to optimize the measurement of epicardial fat. Echocardiography also provides data on traditional cardiac parameters, as well as on left ventricular mass, and diastolic and systolic function, together with the epicardial fat thickness.

Limitations of echocardiographic imaging of epicardial fat Echocardiography may be not the optimal technique for quantification of epicardial fat. Three-dimensional MRI and MDCT are more sensitive and specific than echocardiography for measuring fat thickness in deeper epicardial fat layers in severely obese subjects. Echocardiographic epicardial fat thickness is a linear measurement and therefore may not reflect the total epicardial fat volume in which thickness varies at different locations around the myocardium. MDCT studies found the thickest part of the epicardial fat in the atrioventricular grooves. In addition, epicardial fat is not distributed evenly along the RV free wall. Epicardial fat thickness is usually less in the vicinity of the mid-RV free wall and greater in the distal portion of the RV free wall.

Key points

Echocardiographic epicardial fat thickness is a new, reliable, and simple marker of visceral fat and can be used as a therapeutic target. Echocardiographic epicardial fat thickness cut-off values of 9.5 mm in men and 7.5 mm in women are predictive of metabolic syndrome and high levels of intra-abdominal fat. As echocardiography is routinely performed in obese patients, this objective measure may readily be available at no extra cost. Retrospective reading and analysis of epicardial fat thickness is also possible.

Ultrasound assessment of abdominal fat

Intra-abdominal fat thickness Intra-abdominal fat thickness is defined as the distance between the anterior wall of the aorta and the posterior surface of the rectus abdominis muscle (Figure 5.7).

Intra-abdominal fat thickness is usually measured with a 3.5 or 3.75 MHz probe, 1–5 cm above the umbilicus at the xipho-umbilical line or midway between the xiphoid process and the umbilicus. Intra-abdominal fat thickness correlates with CT visceral fat. A cut-off value of 6.9 cm has been proposed to distinguish between visceral and subcutaneous fat in women.

Limitations of ultrasound assessment of abdominal fat Abdominal imaging is attenuated when the beam travels through 1 cm of fat and the sound level drops by 3 decibels (dB). Thus, in obese patients with large amounts of extra-peritoneal fat, there would be a significant reduction in the original beam intensity or a drop in sound level before the beam enters the peritoneal cavity.

Abdominal wall fat index The abdominal wall fat index is the ratio of maximum preperitoneal to minimum subcutaneous fat thicknesses. An abdominal wall fat index of >1 indicates more prominent visceral adiposity, whereas an index of <1 is suggestive of subcutaneous adiposity.

The abdominal wall fat index can be also used as sonographic index for estimation of regional adiposity. The thicknesses of subcutaneous and preperitoneal fat are measured by placement of a 7.5 or 3.75 MHz

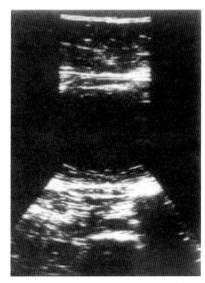

Subcutaneous fat

Intra-abdominal fat

Fig. 5.7 Ultrasonographic intra-abdominal fat thickness. Adapted with permission from Armellini F, Zamboni M, Rigo L, *et al*. (1990) The contribution of sonography to the measurement of intra-abdominal fat. *J Clin Ultrasound* 18:563–7.

probe perpendicular to the skin on the epigastrium. Longitudinal scans are obtained along the middle line. The thickness of the subcutaneous fat is defined as the distance between the anterior surface of the linea alba and the fat–skin barrier. The preperitoneal fat extends from the anterior surface of the liver to the posterior surface of the linea alba. The minimum subcutaneous and maximum preperitoneal fat thicknesses are located immediately below the xiphoid process.

Mesenteric fat thickness

Assessment of mesenteric fat thickness has been also proposed as an index of regional adiposity. Maximal thickness is estimated, and the mean of the three thickest leaves is calculated. This measurement is characterized by good intra-operator and inter-operator reliability.

A cut-off value of 10 mm of mesenteric fat thickness has shown a sensitivity of 70% and a specificity of 75% in differentiating patients with and without metabolic syndrome.

Key points

Ultrasound assessment of intra-abdominal fat is a reproducible and accurate methodology. Among the techniques that are used to assess intra-abdominal fat, ultrasound assessment of intra-abdominal fat thickness seems to be the most reliable index. However, there is no robust evidence that high intra-abdominal fat thickness correlates with high cardiovascular risk, in contrast to the positive relationship shown between echocardiographic epicardial fat thickness and high cardiovascular risk.

Proton magnetic resonance spectroscopy

Intracellular lipid assessment

Proton magnetic resonance spectroscopy (^{1}H-MRS) has been shown to be a valid and reproducible technique for the non-invasive measurement of intra-myocellular and intra-hepatocellular myocardial lipid content in humans. ^{1}H-MRS resolves resonances of various metabolites, including water and fat methyl and methylene groups. The ratio of fat methyl and methylene proton resonance to water proton resonance indicates the fat content relative to that of visible water that can be measured by MRS. The concentration of triglycerides as measured from MRS is calculated based on the assumption that only triglycerides contribute to the lipid signal.

Cardiac ^{1}H-MRS provides sensitive and precise information on the fat tissue content *in vivo*. Localized proton spectroscopy permits the assessment of cardiac fat deposition and myocardial triglyceride levels *in vivo*.

The combination of cardiac and liver imaging methods, as well as MRI, CT, and ultrasound techniques, with ^{1}H-MRS could be a promising tool for estimation of myocardial and liver fat deposition. ^{1}H-MRS examinations are non-invasive and therefore can be repeated many times and with a high temporal resolution.

^{1}H-MRS has the potential to replace biopsy as a follow-up method for intra-myocellular lipid levels.

Key points

¹H-MRS is a valid and reproducible technique for the non-invasive measurement of intracellular lipid content in humans. Its use in clinical practice is desirable.

Dual-energy X-ray absorptiometry

Body fat composition analysis

Dual-energy X-ray absorptiometry (DEXA) is used clinically for whole-body and regional composition analysis. DEXA assesses body composition based on the attenuation of X-rays emitted at two energy levels as they traverse the body.

DEXA provides a definitive method for accurate determination and quantification of fat mass and fat-free mass. DEXA provides less radiation exposure than CT and costs significantly less. A whole-body DEXA scan take between 15 and 35 minutes, depending on the scanner. Measures of total and regional lean mass (coefficient of variation of 1–7%) and fat mass (coefficient of variation of 1–7%) are highly reproducible. DEXA measures of total or appendicular fat and lean mass correlate well with CT or MRI fat measurements. DEXA estimates of intra-abdominal fat are substantially similar to those obtained with waist circumference. The reproducibility of DEXA is around 1.5% for fat.

The application of DEXA to body-composition analysis in obese individuals, as shown in Figure 5.8, is valid, but is subject to practical limitations.

Limitations and advantages of DEXA

The accuracy of DEXA is influenced by several factors in obese subjects. Results may differ depending on several confounding factors such as the scanner model, the software used, and the individual's sagittal diameter and hydration status. DEXA can cause a phenomenon known as 'beam hardening', which may cause the true fat content of obese individuals with a large sagittal diameter to be underestimated.

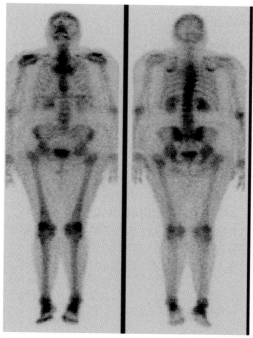

Fig. 5.8 Dual-energy X-ray absorptiometry (DEXA) image of a woman with peripheral obesity.

Hence, adiposity is more likely to be underestimated in the trunk than in the extremities, which have a smaller sagittal diameter.

However, quantitative information on fat mass and fat-free mass can be helpful in assessing and indexing physiological variables as well as metabolic basal rate, insulin sensitivity, and left ventricular mass in obese subjects.

In conclusion, DEXA is a useful tool for assessing total fat mass and lean mass in obese subjects, but can be limited in its ability to measure and discriminate visceral and subcutaneous fat.

Key points

DEXA is a method for quantifying fat mass and fat-free mass. The accuracy and reproducibility of DEXA are influenced by a number of factors in obese subjects. However, the combination of DEXA with an imaging marker of adiposity can provide helpful information in the management of obese subjects.

Bioelectrical impedance

Body fat composition analysis

Bioelectrical impedance (BIA) estimates of body composition are based on the assumption that the overall conductivity of the human body is closely related to lean tissue, which is assumed mostly to be water and conducts the current better than fat. The impedance value is then combined with anthropomorphic data to give body compartment measures.

The use of BIA for body composition analysis in overweight and obese subjects is easy and is largely used in clinical practice. However, only BIA measurements that have been generated recently can provide accurate information on body fat composition. BIA measurements of fat-free mass and fat mass correlate well with DEXA results. BIA measurement can be used to monitor fat and muscle mass changes during weight loss interventions in obese subjects.

Key points

BIA is a non-invasive method for fat and fat-free mass quantification. It is a helpful and practical diagnostic tool for body composition analysis in overweight and obese subjects.

Chapter 6

Echocardiography in obesity

Transthoracic echocardiography in obese subjects

Standard transthoracic echocardiography

Transthoracic echocardiography is an accurate, reliable, non-invasive, and widely used technique to evaluate cardiac morphology and function in obese subjects.

A two-dimensional transthoracic echocardiogram should be carried out as part of the routine assessment of obese subjects in all clinical teaching units, internal medicine wards, and metabolic clinics. Quantitative and qualitative echocardiographic evaluation of cardiovascular function and morphology in obese patients can be considered crucial in stratifying cardiometabolic risk and therefore in deciding on appropriate and effective therapeutic strategies in these subjects.

There is usually no difference in performing and reading a transthoracic echocardiogram between an obese and a non-obese subject. Traditional parasternal long- and short-axis views and an apical view are used to measure echocardiographic parameters in both obese and lean individuals.

Pulsed-wave and continuous-wave Doppler imaging

Pulsed-wave Doppler imaging provides important information regarding flow quantification and timing. Pulsed-wave Doppler signals are transmitted intermittently and received only after a set delay. Its main uses are to determine the pattern of ventricular filling through the mitral valve in diastole, to assess flow patterns in the pulmonary and hepatic veins, and to measure the blood velocity in the LV outflow tract.

Continuous-wave Doppler signals are transmitted and received constantly. They measure frequency shifts along the entire length of the ultrasound beam and are most useful for measuring high velocities. The beam can be steered within the two-dimensional image so that specific areas of the heart can be assessed. The signal can originate from any point along the length of the beam.

The diastolic function of both ventricles in obesity is assessed principally by analysis of pulsed- and continuous-wave Doppler velocity flow profiles at the mitral and tricuspid orifices.

Color Doppler flow imaging

Color flow mapping superimposes multiple pulsed-wave Doppler signals onto the two-dimensional echocardiographic image and ascribes a color code to each velocity. Normal blood flow is laminar and is shown in a uniform color, with red conventionally coding for blood flow towards the transducer, and blue for blood flow away. When blood flow exceeds this threshold, it results in 'aliasing', whereby a reversal of colors occurs. Turbulent flow induces a range of velocities. The clinical applications of color Doppler imaging are similar in obese and non-obese individuals.

Tissue Doppler imaging

Tissue Doppler imaging (TDI) is a relatively new echocardiographic technique that uses Doppler principles to measure the velocity of myocardial motion. TDI can be performed in pulsed-wave and color modes. Pulsed-wave TDI is used to measure peak myocardial velocities and is particularly well suited to the measurement of long-axis ventricular motion. Because the apex remains relatively stationary throughout the cardiac cycle, mitral annular motion is a good surrogate measure of overall longitudinal LV contraction and relaxation. To measure longitudinal myocardial velocities, the sample volume is placed in the ventricular myocardium immediately adjacent to the mitral annulus. The cardiac cycle is represented by three waveforms: S, systolic myocardial velocity above the baseline as the annulus descends towards the apex; E, early diastolic myocardial relaxation velocity below the baseline as the annulus ascends away

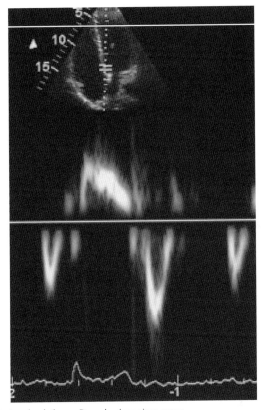

Fig. 6.1 A standard tissue Doppler imaging curve.

from the apex; and A, myocardial velocity associated with atrial contraction, as depicted in a standard TDI curve (Figure 6.1) in a normoweight subject.

Strain rate imaging

The concept of regional myocardial strain can be defined as fractional tissue deformation in response to an applied force (stress). Strain rate imaging (SRI) is a new echocardiographic TDI-derived technique that can provide data on regional myocardial function. Regional deformation (strain) and deformation rate (strain rate) can be calculated non-invasively in both the LV and right ventricle (RV), providing information on regional LV dysfunction.

Both TDI and SRI can show early obesity-related functional changes, particularly diastolic and systolic changes, that cannot be detected by conventional echocardiography.

Contrast echocardiography

Contrast echocardiography can improve the diagnostic accuracy of technically suboptimal studies when used in conjunction with harmonic imaging in obese patients with limited transthoracic windows. Intravenous ultrasound contrast agents are indicated for LV opacification and improvement of LV endocardial border delineation in patients with suboptimal acoustic windows. Its application in clinical practice is still not used worldwide. However, its use may be suggested in severely obese subjects with poor transthoracic windows.

Limitations of transthoracic echocardiography in obese subjects

Echocardiographic assessment of extremely obese patients can sometimes be limited by technical factors. Firstly, ergonomics factors should be considered. Echocardiographic beds should be able to accommodate severely obese subjects and should therefore have adequate weight capacity. This can represent a practical problem in some institutions. In some obese subjects with severe obstructive pulmonary disease, the high echocardiographic impedance due to the lung hyperinflation may not allow an accurate view and reliable reading from the parasternal views. In these cases, a subcostal view may help and should therefore be suggested. However, subcostal imaging in obese patients with severe obstructive pulmonary disease, whilst certainly helpful, is usually very difficult in obese patients with large abdomens. In severely obese individuals, the heart can assume a horizontal position in the mediastinum. This may produce anterior and rightward displacement of the RV, and posterior and lateral displacement of the LV. Scanning from the base to the apex of the heart may require a horizontal sweep rather than the usual inferior and lateral angulation. Right heart structure and function measurement can be challenging in obese subjects.

Transesophageal echocardiography in obese subjects

Transesophageal echocardiography provides excellent visualization of cardiac structures. Transesophageal echocardiography is particularly indicated for investigation of valvular heart disease, aortic diseases, endocarditis, and intracardiac and extracardiac masses including pulmonary embolism, and for evaluation of patent foramen ovale and its association with central and peripheral embolic events. Transesophageal echocardiography has a major role as a diagnostic tool in several clinical scenarios. Conditions and settings in which transesophageal echocardiography provides the most definitive diagnosis are hemodynamically unstable patients with suboptimal transthoracic images or patients with suspected aortic dissection or aortic injury and other conditions in which transesophageal echocardiography is superior to transthoracic echocardiography, as well as suspected endocarditis and a cardiac or aortic source of emboli.

Limitations of transesophageal echocardiography in obese subjects

The safety, practicability, and limitations of transesophageal echocardiography in obese subjects must be considered. Minor complications occur with equal frequency in obese and normoweight subjects. However, morbidly obese patients may present transient oxygen desaturation during upper gastrointestinal endoscopy more commonly than normoweight subjects. Transient hypotension is lower in obesity, whereas the incidence of transient hypertension can be slightly higher in obese subjects compared with normoweight subjects. The conclusion is that transesophageal echocardiography can be performed safely in patients who are obese. However, proper precautions must be taken, as well as the routine use of supplementary oxygen in morbidly obese subjects with or without obstructive sleep apnea.

Echocardiographic morphological changes in obese subjects

Left ventricular mass

Increased LV mass (LVM) is a well-recognized and independent cardiovascular risk factor. Increased LVM can be predictive of cardiovascular events and therefore LVM can be targeted during medical interventions in obesity. LVM is now routinely assessed by echocardiography. Echocardiographic LVM can be calculated from M-mode measurements (Box 6.1) or from two-dimensional volumetric models (see Figure 6.2). Both methods have been validated by estimation of human LVM at autopsy and so have become widely used.

Box 6.1 Left ventricular mass calculations from M-mode measurement

$$\text{LVM (Penn)} = 1.04 \times [(\text{LVIDD} + \text{PWTD} + \text{IVSTD})^3$$
$$- \text{LVIDD}^3] - 13.6 \text{ g}$$
$$\text{LVM (ASE)} = 0.8 \times [1.04(\text{LVIDD} + \text{PWTD} + \text{IVSTD})^3$$
$$- \text{LVIDD}^3)] + 0.6 \text{ g}$$

where LVIDD is left ventricular internal diameter in diastole, PWTD is posterior wall thickness in diastole and IVSTD is interventricular septum thickness in diastole (all in mm).

Penn, Penn Convention; ASE, American Society of Echocardiography.

LVM can be calculated from two-dimensional linear LV measurements. The most commonly used two-dimensional methods for measuring LVM are based on the area–length formula and the truncated ellipsoid model. Both methods rely on measurements of myocardial area at the mid-papillary muscle level. LVM can be estimated from short-axis (Figure 6.2, left) and apical four-chamber (Figure 6.2, right) two-dimensional echo views using the area–length formula or the truncated ellipsoid formula.

Indexing left ventricular mass in obese subjects

Careful attention is required for correct LVM interpretation in obese subjects. The absolute value of LVM, which is often the only measure taken, is often higher in obese patients than in lean subjects; however, physiological and anthropometric factors, as well as body surface area

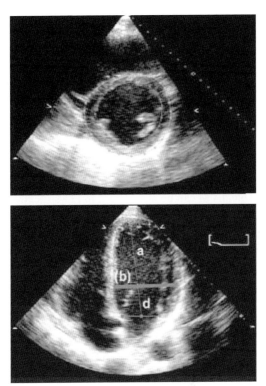

Fig. 6.2 Two methods for estimating left ventricular mass based on area–length formula and the truncated ellipsoid formula, from short-axis (top) and apical four-chamber (bottom) two-dimensional echo views. In the right panel, 'a' is the long or semi-major axis from the widest minor axis radius to the apex, 'b' is the short-axis radius (backcalculated from the short-axis cavity area), and 'd' is the truncated semi-major axis from widest short-axis diameter to the mitral anulus plane. Reproduced from: Lang RM, Bierig M, Devereux RB, *et al.* (2005) Recommendations for Chamber Quantification: A Report from the American Society of Echocardiography's Guidelines and Standards Committee and the Chamber Quantification Writing Group, developed in conjunction with the European Association of Echocardiography, a branch of the European Society of Cardiology. *J Am Soc Echocardiogr* 18:1440–63, with permission from Elsevier.

(BSA) and height, have to be considered when LVM is measured. Additionally, because both fat mass (FM) and free-fat mass (FFM) are usually increased in obese individuals, LVM needs to be adjusted to obtain an appropriate measurement.

Indexed LVM values should be considered in obese subjects. LVM may be adjusted for BSA, height (h), height$^{2.7}$ (h$^{2.7}$) or FFM in kg of body weight (FMM$_{kg}$).

To correctly evaluate LVM in obese subjects, it has been suggested that indexing LVM to h$^{2.7}$ may be more appropriate than normalization to BSA or even height. Where regional body fat distribution analysis is available, LVM can be normalized to FFM$_{kg}$. Extremely obese patients exhibit greater FM than FFM; therefore, it can be assumed that LVM is likely to be more strongly related to FFM than to adipose mass. Thus, by indexing LVM to FFM$_{kg}$, the confounding effect of higher FFM on LVM in severely obese subjects can be excluded. Interestingly, after indexing by lean body mass, there are no gender differences in LVM, and the relative effects of adiposity and blood pressure appear to be of similar magnitude.

LVM/h$^{2.7}$ or LVM/FFM$_{kg}$ is the most appropriate index for LVM quantification in obese populations. In clinical practice, LVM/h$^{2.7}$ is the easiest parameter for LVM estimation and is therefore most often recommended.

LVM/h$^{2.7}$ is commonly higher in morbidly obese subjects when compared with lean individuals. However, LVM/h$^{2.7}$ is not statistically different between metabolically healthy but obese (MHO) and lean subjects, as shown in Table 6.1. MHO subjects are individuals

Table 6.1 Indexed left ventricle mass (LVM) in a sample of morbidly obese, metabolically healthy but obese (MHO), and lean subjects

Subject	LVM (g/h$^{2.7}$)
Morbidly obese	60±10*
MHO	45±10
Lean	40±10

* Significantly different from lean subjects ($P<0.01$).

Adapted with permission from Iacobellis G, *et al.* (2002) Influence of excess fat on cardiac morphology and function: study in uncomplicated obesity. *Obes Res* 10:767–73.

who are obese, but free of common obesity-related complications (see Chapter 3).

> ## Key points
>
> $LVM/h^{2.7}$ is the most commonly used and the most appropriate index for correct LVM quantification in obese subjects. $LVM/h^{2.7}$ is commonly higher in morbidly obese people, but may not differ significantly between MHO and lean subjects.

Appropriateness of left ventricle mass in obese subjects

Obesity—both complicated and uncomplicated—is commonly associated with LV remodeling or abnormal geometry. This remodeling can be appropriate or inappropriate. The concept of inappropriate LVM can be explained by an increase in LVM higher than necessary to compensate for the increased workload. Inappropriate LVM has been reported to be associated mainly with concentric geometry.

MHO subjects can present with normal LVM or appropriate LVH, particularly appropriate eccentric LVH, as reported in Table 6.2. It has been suggested that adaptive mechanisms can occur in MHO subjects. However, maladaptive and inappropriate LV geometric patterns can develop also in MHO subjects. Inappropriate concentric LV hypertrophy seems to be the most common type of maladaptive LV

Table 6.2 Left ventricle (LV) geometry and appropriateness of LV mass (LVM) in a population of metabolically healthy but obese subjects

LV geometry	Appropriate LVM (%)	Inappropriate LVM (%)
No LVH	55	0
Eccentric LVH	22	10
Concentric LVH	0	18
Concentric remodeling	0	5

LVH, LV hypertrophy.

Adapted with permission from Iacobellis G, Ribaudo MC, Zappaterreno A, Iannucci CV, Di Mario U & Leonetti F (2004) Adapted changes in left ventricular structure and function in severe uncomplicated obesity. *Obes Res* 12:1616–21.

remodeling in MHO subjects (Table 6.2). Concentric LV remodeling, characterized by an increase in the relative wall thickness and normal LVM, or eccentric LV hypertrophy can be observed also in normotensive, non-diabetic, obese subjects. Whether this maladaptive mechanism is a natural consequence of long-term obesity or is due to the occurrence of obesity-related subclinical abnormalities is still unclear.

Left ventricular geometry in obese subjects

Hypertrophy is a compensatory remodeling of the LV in response to pressure or volume overload. Obesity, particularly when complicated by hypertension and diabetes, can be associated with LV hypertrophy (LVH). Transthoracic two-dimensional echocardiography is undoubtedly the most used and reliable method to estimate LVH in obese subjects. Measurements for LVH quantification can be obtained from standard two-dimensional and mono-dimensional parasternal long- and short-axis views.

Several echocardiographic cut-off points for LVH have been proposed. In general, LVH is defined as LVM/BSA of ≥ 134 g/m^2 for men and ≥ 110 g/m^2 for women, and as LVM/h$^{2.7}$ of ≥ 51 g/m$^{2.7}$ in both genders. LVM/h$^{2.7}$ is highly recommended for a correct LVH estimation in obese patients. Threshold values for LVH calculated as LVM/FFM$_{kg}$ are still under development.

Four LV geometric patterns (normal, concentric remodeling, concentric hypertrophy, and eccentric hypertrophy) can be found in obese subjects, as summarized in Box 6.2.

Box 6.2 Echocardiographic LV geometric patterns

- Normal (no LVH and RWT ≤ 0.44)
- Concentric remodeling (no LVH and RWT ≥ 0.44)
- Concentric hypertrophy (LVH and RWT ≥ 0.44)
- Eccentric hypertrophy (LVH and RWT ≤ 0.44).

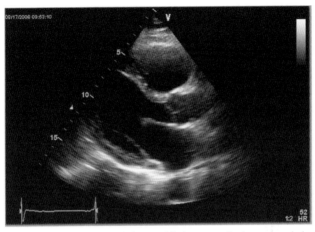

Fig. 6.3 Appropriate eccentric left ventricle hypertrophy in a severely but uncomplicated obese subject: parasternal long-axis view. Image from the author's collection.

Relative wall thickness (RWT) is required to evaluate LV geometry in obese subjects who undergo a transthoracic echocardiogram. RWT is calculated as 2 × LV posterior wall/LV end-diastolic diameter.

Uncomplicated obesity can be associated with normal LV geometry or with appropriate eccentric LVH (Figure 6.3). Complicated obesity is frequently associated with appropriate or inappropriate LVH, mostly of concentric (Figure 6.4) and eccentric patterns.

Other left ventricle parameters

LV diameters and wall thickness are routinely measured from M-mode tracing or using digital calipers to perform point-to-point assessment from two-dimensional images. LV volumes are usually calculated using a modified Simpson's biplane method.

Obesity is frequently associated with increased interventricular septum and posterior wall thickness (PWS), enlarged LV end-diastolic diameter (LVEDD) and LV elevated end-diastolic volume (LVEDV). End diastole is defined as the start of the QRS complex on an electrocardiogram tracing. However, as for LVM, these parameters may be normal in MHO subjects when compared with normoweight subjects.

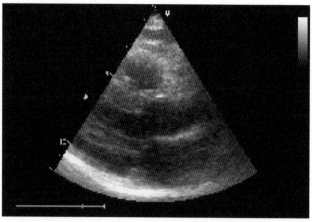

Fig. 6.4 Concentric left ventricle hypertrophy in a morbid hypertensive obese subject: parasternal long-axis view. Image from the author's collection.

The left atrium in obese subjects

Echocardiographic left atrium (LA) measurements are very important in obese subjects. A standard echocardiogram can provide linear LA measurements, as well as area and volume. LA can be measured at ventricular end systole from M-mode tracing. Linear LA dimensions can be obtained from the parasternal long-axis view at the aortic cusp level. LA area and volume can be calculated from an apical four-chamber view. LA volume determination is preferred over linear dimensions because it allows accurate assessment of the asymmetric remodeling of the LA chamber.

LA volume is measured using the biplane area–length method. Apical four- and two-chamber views for determination of LA area are obtained and the length from the center of the plane of the mitral annulus to the posterior wall is considered. If the LA in the two-chamber view is foreshortened, the apical long-axis view is used. The maximal LA chamber area and length are measured at the end of ventricular systole. LA volume is calculated from the formula $(0.85 \times A1 \times A2)/L$, where A1 is the four-chamber LA area, A2 is the two-chamber or apical long-axis LA area, and L is the smallest of the two lengths obtained.

Table 6.3 Left atrium (LA) dimensions in a sample of morbidly obese, metabolically healthy but obese (MHO), and lean subjects

Subject	LA dimension (cm)
Morbidly obese	4.3±0.5*
MHO	3.7±0.5
Lean	3.2±0.5

LA dimensions indicate the M-mode linear dimension obtained from the parasternal long-axis view.

* Significantly different from lean subjects ($P<0.01$).

Adapted from Iacobellis G, et al. (2002) Influence of excess fat on cardiac morphology and function: study in uncomplicated obesity. Obes Res 10:767–73.

LA dimensions, volume, and areas are usually higher in obese than in normoweight subjects. LA enlargement has been described in both morbidly obese and MHO subjects (Table 6.3). The need to normalize LA dimensions for differences in body size in obese subjects remain the subject of discussion. As recently suggested, LA normalization using body weight, height, FFM or BSA, as optimal allometric exponents, seems to remove the effect of body size. BSA accounts for variations in body size and should therefore be used to normalize LA diameter and volume.

The aortic root in obese subjects

Aortic root measurements can be obtained from a two-dimensional parasternal long-axis view or more commonly from M-mode tracing. The root is measured at the cuspal level. Echocardiographic aortic root dimension is frequently higher in obese subjects, both morbidly obese and MHO subjects. Aortic stiffness can be altered in obese subjects.

The right ventricle in obese subjects

As for the LV chambers, the RV cavity and wall thickness can be calculated using a conventional echocardiogram in obese subjects. RV parameters are preferably measured using point-to-point assessment from two-dimensional images.

RV end-diastolic diameter and RV end-systolic diameter are commonly found to be greater in obese subjects, particularly in patients with obstructive sleep apnea (OSA), increased visceral adiposity, and insulin resistance. Echocardiographic RV measurement in obese subjects can be useful as a diagnostic marker and therapeutic target in severely obese subjects affected by OSA.

The pulmonary artery in obese subjects

The increased pulmonary blood volume associated with the increased total blood volume in morbidly obese subjects increases the pulmonary artery pressure and pulmonary vascular resistance. Pulmonary artery dimensions may also be increased in obese subjects, particularly in morbidly obese subjects with OSA. Pulmonary artery measurements can be obtained by point-to-point assessment from a two-dimensional parasternal short-axis view at the aortic valve level. Pulmonary artery pressure can be estimated accurately and noninvasively by using continuous-wave Doppler ultrasound measurement of the peak velocity of a tricuspid regurgitant jet. However, it is often difficult to obtain adequate tricuspid regurgitation signals for measurement of pulmonary artery pressure.

Peak RV systolic pressure is also commonly used to estimate pulmonary artery pressure in obese patients. The maximum peak tricuspid regurgitation velocity recorded with continuous-wave Doppler imaging is used to determine the RV systolic pressure, with right atrial pressure assumed to be 10 mmHg. Pulmonary artery pressure is assumed to equate to RV systolic pressure in the absence of pulmonary stenosis and RV outflow tract obstruction. Obese individuals may present with an RV systolic pressure of 35 mmHg or more.

Non-invasive determination of pulmonary pressure is possible using TDI. TDI is useful in determining the mechanical properties of RV function in obese patients with pulmonary hypertension. The isovolumic relaxation time of the RV free wall measured by pulsed TDI, the systolic velocity of the tricuspid valve annulus obtained by pulsed TDI, and tricuspid annular plane systolic excursion by two-dimensional echocardiography can be used to estimate pulmonary artery pressure. Peak systolic velocity and strain correlate with pulmonary hemodynamics. RV myocardial strain also seems to correlate significantly with pulmonary hemodynamics in patients with pulmonary hypertension and normal LV function.

Echocardiographic functional changes in obesity
Systole in obese subjects

Results of studies evaluating LV systolic function in obese subjects have largely produced controversial results. Some studies have shown that obese subjects have preserved LV systolic function or hyperdynamic systole, whereas others have demonstrated subclinical and regional systolic dysfunction.

Hyperdynamic systole is usually defined by an ejection fraction (EF) higher than 75%, whereas an EF between 55 and 75% suggests preserved or normal LV systole. The discrepancies in LV systolic function are mostly due to the presence or absence of obesity-related complications and to the different echocardiographic techniques used to estimate LV systole. Conventional echocardiographic measures such as EF, fractional shortening, and circumferential fiber shortening are considered relatively insensitive methods; however, the newer echo techniques can detect subclinical LV functional changes.

LV systole in obese subjects by conventional echocardiography

LV systolic function can be estimated by endocardial and mid-wall indices: EF is calculated using Simpson's ellipsoid, which estimates LV volumes; fractional shortening (FS) at the endocardium is calculated by using the formula FS = (LVEDD – LVIDD)/LVEDD; and mid-wall shortening (MWS) is estimated after taking into account the epicardial migration of the mid-wall during systole using a modified ellipsoidal model. Circumferential end-systolic stress (cESS) is calculated at the mid-wall at the level of the LV minor axis, as a measure of myocardial afterload. Myocardial contractility can be estimated by expressing MWS as a percentage of the value for a given cESS (cMWS). Meridional ESS (mESS) is also used as measure of afterload, calculated using the formula 333 × (systolic blood pressure × LVESD)/[posterior wall thickness × (1 + posterior wall thickness/LVESD)], where LVESD is LV end-systolic diameter. LV stroke volume and systemic output (LV stroke volume × heart rate) are also common systole parameters that can be measured by standard echocardiography in obese subjects. FS, EF, MWS, and cMWS may be the same or higher and therefore supranormal in obese patients when compared with lean subjects.

LV systole in obese subjects by TDI

The M-mode calculations for FS, MWS, and mESS are actually rarely used in routine practice and have now largely been superseded by TDI data. TDI of mitral motion can provide information about LV regional myocardial motion in obese subjects. Mitral annular motion is a good surrogate measure of overall longitudinal LV contraction.

Global systolic LV longitudinal function assessed by TDI is estimated by S-wave peak velocities (Sm global). Results on global systolic myocardial velocity in obesity are controversial. The global S-wave peak has been found to be normal or lower in obese subjects when compared with lean subjects. Systolic peak velocity at the lateral wall level may be lower in obese subjects than in normoweight subjects. Impaired global or segmental systolic myocardial velocity can suggest subclinical LV systolic dysfunction in obese subjects, even when EF is preserved.

LV systole in obese subjects by SRI

Regional myocardial velocity and strain/strain rate can be assessed by SRI in obese subjects. Subclinical systolic dysfunction in obese subjects can also be estimated with SRI.

Measurement of regional strain rate and strain can be performed in either the longitudinal or the radial direction for each myocardial segment, and each direction reflects different aspects of regional myocardial function. However, this new technique may be limited by the fact that analysis of tissue velocities, strain and strain rate by SRI is angle-dependent.

Systolic strain and systolic strain rate, which indicate regional myocardial longitudinal deformation, both at the septum and at the lateral wall levels, are usually impaired in obese patients. In fact, the regional myocardial systolic strain findings evaluated either at the medium septal or at the lateral wall level are significantly lower in obese patients when compared with normoweight subjects. The regional myocardial systolic strain rate, at both the medium septal and lateral walls, is also usually lower in obese patients than in non-obese individuals.

RV function

Increases in pulmonary artery pressure and pulmonary vascular resistance in morbidly obese patients may result in increased RV afterload.

Thus, morbidly obese subjects may develop RV dysfunction as a result of the increased RV afterload.

The RV performance index (Tei index) has been calculated and validated using TDI-derived, rather than conventional, pulsed Doppler time intervals. RV TDI indices have been shown to be useful in the detection of subclinical and clinical disease in morbid obesity and in chronic pulmonary and systemic disease. TDI-derived RV strain imaging can detect segmental myocardial dysfunction, overcoming the limitations of conventional TDI resulting from tethering.

Key points

LV systole assessed by conventional echocardiography in obese subjects can be hyperdynamic, as defined by an EF of $\geq 75\%$. However, TDI and SRI detect subclinical regional LV systolic abnormalities in obese subjects. Whilst global systolic LV longitudinal function can be preserved in obese subjects, regional myocardial longitudinal deformation is usually impaired in these subjects.

Diastole in obese subjects

Obese patients commonly display features of diastolic dysfunction. Diastolic dysfunction affects both morbidly and MHO subjects, and is characterized either by early impairment of LV relaxation or by increased myocardial stiffness. RV-impaired diastole is also frequently observed in obese subjects.

LV diastole in obese subjects by conventional echocardiography

LV diastolic function can be evaluated using the following pulsed-wave Doppler echocardiographic parameters. Pulsed-wave Doppler flow pattern at the mitral anulus is traced electronically to measure peak velocities of early and late diastolic LV filling: early (E) and late (A) transmitral peak flow velocities, as well as the E/A ratio, indicating the pattern of LV diastolic filling. Isovolumic relaxation time (IVRT) is measured between the end of transaortic systolic flow (outflow) and the beginning of the E wave (inflow), identified using color continuos-wave

Doppler across the LV inflow outflow pattern and placing the pulsed-wave Doppler beam close to the anterior mitral valve leaflet.

The pulse wave of pulmonary vein flow into the LA can be also calculated and indicates LV filling pressure. S, D, and A waves represent systolic and diastolic LV filling. A pulmonary A wave duration 30 ms greater than the transmitral A wave could suggest high LV filling pressure. Obese subjects affected by OSA can show this pattern.

The commonest echocardiographic findings of diastolic dysfunction in obese subjects are a decreased E/A ratio, prolongation of IVRT, and deceleration time of early diastolic mitral flow (DTE).

LV filling is indicated by E/A ratio, IVRT can be considered a marker of LV relaxation, and DTE can be used as an index of LV stiffness, as summarized in Table 6.4. The delayed diastolic filling and prolonged LV relaxation may induce progressive enlargement of the LA.

LV diastole in obese subjects by TDI

TDI can provide useful and accurate information about early LV diastolic filling and relaxation abnormalities in obese subjects. TDI provides an assessment of LV relaxation and, in combination with conventional Doppler measurements, allows non-invasive estimation of LV filling pressure. Pulsed-wave TDI of the septal annulus is used for measurements of early peak diastolic mitral annulus velocity (Es). LV filling pressures are approximated from the relationship of E/Es (E being derived by mitral flow velocity).

In obese subjects, all diastolic phases are altered according to TDI parameters. Es and myocardial diastolic velocity are reduced and LV filling pressure, approximated by the E/Es ratio, is increased.

Table 6.4 Conventional diastolic parameters in a sample of obese and lean subjects

	Obese	Lean	*P* value
E/A ratio	1.4±0.5	2±0.5	≤0.01
IVRT	120±10.	90±10	≤0.01
DTE	210±10	180±10	≤0.01

E/A ratio, early/late transmitral peak flow velocities ratio; IVRT, isovolumic relaxation time; DTE, deceleration time of early diastolic mitral flow.

Adapted with permission from Iacobellis G, *et al.* (2002) Influence of excess fat on cardiac morphology and function: study in uncomplicated obesity. *Obes Res* 10:767–73.

Regional diastolic function detected at the medium septum and the lateral wall levels is also impaired in obese subjects.

Early diastolic myocardial velocity (Em global), assessed by TDI, is generally lower in obese subjects when compared with lean subjects, suggesting subclinical diastolic dysfunction. Late diastolic peak velocity, IVRT sampled at the septum annular level, and E/Es ratio, both at the septum and the lateral wall level, are all usually higher in obese compared with normoweight subjects.

RV diastole in obese subjects by conventional echocardiography

Obese subjects frequently have abnormal echocardiographic diastole parameters indicating an impaired diastolic filling and relaxation, and stiffness.

RV diastole in obese subjects by TDI

TDI of the RV in clinical practice is relatively limited. However, its use may be of help in the assessment of RV function in obese patients. TDI may detect subclinical RV dysfunction associated with obesity, even when two-dimensional echocardiographic assessment of RV function is normal.

Obese subjects with a body mass index (BMI) >35 kg/m^2 may have reduced RV function compared with controls, as shown by lower myocardial velocities during systole (Sa) and early diastole (Ea), peak RV strain, and peak RV strain rate. RV Ea is significantly lower in obese but otherwise healthy patients compared with controls, despite normal global RV function using conventional parameters in both groups. RV Sa and Ea increase significantly following bariatric surgery weight loss.

Key points

Obesity is characterized by diastolic dysfunction, which is routinely assessed by conventional and TDI echocardiography. LV diastolic filling, relaxation, and stiffness can all be abnormal in obese subjects, and global and regional diastolic functions are impaired. The E/A ratio and early diastolic myocardial velocity are usually lower in obese compared with normoweight subjects. LV filling pressure, approximated by the E/Es ratio, is increased in obese individuals.

Myocardial performance index

The myocardial performance index (MPI) is a Doppler-derived index that reflects LV systolic and diastolic function. MPI is defined as IVRT plus the isovolumic contraction time (IVCT) divided by the LV ejection time (ET). MPI is calculated using the formula MPI = (R–R interval – mitral inflow time – ET)/ET, where R–R interval is the interval between R waves. MPI has been described as being higher in obese women, but its interpretation can be affected by the increased preload and heart rate variability associated with obesity. MPI may have limited use in obese subjects without cardiovascular disease. Further studies will be necessary to test its utility in obese populations.

Echocardiographic myocardial texture analysis in obese subjects

The myocardial texture and function of severely obese patients can be evaluated using ultrasonic integrated backscatter (IBS) analysis. The quantitative IBS signal is thought to be directly related to myocardial collagen content, one of the primary determinants of myocardial reflectivity. The images are obtained using harmonic imaging mode.

A cyclic variation index of both septum and posterior wall levels, and IBS variations of both septum and posterior wall, have been described as significantly lower in obese compared with normoweight subjects, whereas IBS_{si} (IBS at the septum level) and the mean (IBS_{msi}) (expressed as a percentage) are significantly higher in obese than in non-obese individuals.

These findings may suggest subclinical impaired myocardial intrinsic contractility and increased myocardial reflectivity in obese subjects. Although promising and of great interest, further studies will be necessary before IBS can be performed routinely in all obese subjects.

Echocardiographic changes in metabolically healthy but obese subjects

Some of the echocardiographic changes that have been reported and described in this chapter are commonly observed in obese subjects. However, it is sometimes difficult to discriminate the effect of obesity

Box 6.3 Morphological and functional cardiac changes in MHO subjects

- Normal LV mass
- Appropriate eccentric LV hypertrophy (mostly in subjects with a BMI >50 kg/m^2)
- Inappropriate concentric LV hypertrophy (mostly in subjects with a BMI >50 kg/m^2)
- Increased RV mass (mostly in subjects with a BMI >50 kg/m^2)
- Increased LA size
- Aortic root enlargement
- Hyperdynamic or preserved systole
- Normal global LV contractility
- Subclinical regional myocardial dysfunction
- Normal or lower-end and circumferential systolic stress
- Global and segmental diastolic dysfunction
- Increased LV filling pressure
- Impaired LV and RV diastolic filling
- Impaired LV and RV diastolic relaxation.

by itself and of obesity-related complications, even those that are sub-clinical, on the echocardiographic parameters. Uncomplicated metabolically healthy obesity is associated with more functional adaptive or subclinical changes than morphological abnormalities. These are summarized in Box 6.3.

Echocardiographic epicardial fat thickness

Epicardial fat thickness is measured from parasternal long- and short-axis views and usually appears as the echo-free space between the outer wall of the myocardium and the visceral layer of pericardium (Figure 6.5).

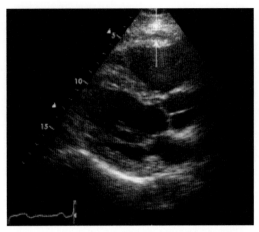

Fig. 6.5 Echocardiographic epicardial fat thickness. Image from the author's collection.

Echocardiographic epicardial fat thickness range varies from a minimum of 1 mm to a maximum observed value of 25 mm. Echocardiography shows that the higher the epicardial fat thickness, the higher the LVM in obese subjects, independent of blood pressure values. Epicardial fat is also related to diastolic dysfunction, commonly observed in obese subjects.

Key points

Epicardial fat is identified as the echo-free space between the outer wall of the myocardium and the visceral layer of pericardium. High echocardiographic epicardial fat thickness is associated with high LVM, abnormal LV geometry, and impaired diastolic function in obese subjects.

Chapter 7

Obesity and atherosclerosis

Atherosclerosis

Atherosclerosis is a disease of the large- and medium-sized arteries characterized by a gradual build-up of fatty and inflammatory plaques within the arterial wall, which may eventually result in a significant reduction in the vessel lumen, impairing blood flow and perfusion to the distal tissues including the heart and the brain. These fatty plaques may also become vulnerable and unstable and then trigger thrombosis. Major clinical complications of atherosclerosis are coronary artery disease and stroke.

Obesity and coronary artery disease

Coronary artery disease is a complex disease characterized by narrowing or blockage of the coronary arteries, usually caused by atherosclerosis. Coronary artery disease is the most common type of heart disease, including myocardial infarction and angina pectoris. It is the leading cause of death in both men and women. Obesity is a major, but modifiable, risk factor. The influence of excess body weight on the development of coronary artery disease has been assessed largely by numerous epidemiological prospective and observational studies. The risk of developing coronary artery disease associated with overweight and obesity increases substantially with exposure to other atherosclerotic risk factors. Nevertheless, the association between obesity and overall mortality and cardiovascular events in patients with coronary artery disease is controversial. Many studies have found a clear correlation between obesity and coronary artery disease, whilst others have not.

The association between body mass index (BMI) and acute coronary syndrome, defined as a diagnosis of unstable angina or acute myocardial infarction, has been always considered strong and independent.

However, there is much scientific and clinical debate on how obesity is currently measured and which indices are currently used. The main research and clinical evidence-based opinions suggest that the risk of coronary artery disease should be based on regional fat distribution rather than overall obesity as expressed by BMI. In fact, robust evidence now shows that abdominal central adiposity should be considered the best independent predictor of myocardial infarction rather than overall obesity. Recent large epidemiological trials have clearly indicated that abdominal visceral obesity is one of the major risk factors for coronary artery disease across all ethnic groups—subjects who present excess visceral abdominal truncal fat are more prone to develop coronary artery disease than subjects with prevalent subcutaneous obesity.

Increased waist circumference is particularly associated with an increased risk of myocardial infarction in men, and increased waist-to-hip ratio (WHR) is associated with an increased risk of myocardial infarction, cardiovascular death, and stroke in women.

When compared with normoweight or underweight subjects, obese patients with a BMI of 30–35 kg/m^2 have no increased risk for total mortality or cardiovascular mortality for coronary artery disease. In contrast, a low BMI is strongly associated with an increased long-term risk of total mortality and other cardiovascular events.

Some protective effect of the adipose tissue, particularly the subcutaneous fat depot, on coronary arteries has been suggested. The adipose tissue may also change its metabolic and biochemical properties in response to atherosclerotic injuries through adaptive hormonal and hemodynamic mechanisms. However, it should also be noted that these obese patients are generally younger and with a higher percentage of single vessel disease, which may also impact on mortality and morbidity.

With regard to cardiovascular outcomes following cardiac interventions, the role of obesity based on BMI has recently been revised. It has been suggested that BMI-defined obesity is not associated with increased mortality and morbidity following coronary revascularization. Obese patients with unstable angina or non-ST-elevation myocardial infarction who are treated with early revascularization may have less long-term mortality than normoweight patients. A short-term protective effect of a higher BMI in patients undergoing percutaneous transluminal coronary angioplasty has been also reported.

It has been speculated that obese patients with a better short- to medium-term outcome after coronary revascularization may present some resistance to ischemia–reperfusion injury. Increase adiponectin production after coronary revascularization has been evoked as one of the potential protective mechanisms. The inability of BMI to discriminate between an excess of body fat and lean mass is a possible explanation of the better outcomes in overweight and mildly obese patients.

Nevertheless, given the fact that results are still partially contradictory, excess adiposity as measured by BMI may be still associated with an increased risk of coronary artery disease and with recurrent coronary events following acute myocardial infarction. This seems to be true particularly among those who are obese and survive to hospital discharge following the first acute myocardial infarction. This finding may be also associated with the absence of or inadequate coronary revascularization and inappropriate secondary or tertiary preventive treatment after the myocardial infarction. Obesity-related comorbidities, as well as diabetes and hypertension, older age, smoking, and different ethnicities, can increase the risk of coronary artery disease and so negatively impact on cardiovascular outcomes.

In addition, obese patients appear to have reduced collateral vessel development. However, appropriate angiographic imaging is necessary to estimate the degree of collateralization. Image quality can be affected by the thickness of the chest wall and so may lead to an underestimation of collateral vessel development in obese subjects.

Key points

Visceral adiposity is a major predictor of coronary artery disease. Abdominal central fat accumulation predicts the risk of myocardial infarction better than overall obesity. Subjects who present excess visceral abdominal truncal fat are more prone to develop coronary artery disease than subjects with prevalent subcutaneous obesity. By contrast, increased BMI seems to provide a better outcome in individuals who undergo coronary revascularization interventions. Waist circumference or other markers of visceral fatness may be more helpful than BMI in predicting and stratifying coronary artery disease risk in overweight or obese patients.

Obesity and stroke

Morbid obesity is a risk factor for stroke. The effect of obesity-related hypertension, diabetes, and hyperlipidemia on stroke has been well documented. However, evidence for an association between obesity alone and the risk of stroke is weak.

Two large epidemiological studies looked at the impact of morbid obesity on the development and progression of stroke. In a prospective Physicians' Health Study in 2005, patients with a BMI of 25–30 and >30 kg/m^2 had a higher adjusted relative risk of total stroke compared with men with a BMI of <25 kg/m^2. With each one-unit increase in BMI score, the multiple adjusted rate of ischemic stroke increased by 4% and of hemorrhagic stroke by 6%. Fatal and non-fatal incidences of stroke were recorded by using the Swedish National Register on Cause of Death and the Swedish Hospital Discharge Registry. According to the results of the Health Study, men who started the study with a BMI of between 20 and 22.49 kg/m^2 were significantly less likely to suffer a stroke than those who started with a BMI >30 kg/m^2. However, no significant association was found between BMI and risk of hemorrhagic stroke.

Both increased BMI and WHR have been reported to be independent risk factors for stroke, even after adjusting for hypertension, hypercholesterolemia, and diabetes. However, abdominal obesity may be more closely related to stroke risk. The association of BMI and abdominal obesity (WHR) with stroke incidence was examined in a large number of male health professionals, aged 40–75 years, who had no history of cardiovascular disease or stroke. Compared with men in the lowest quintile of BMI, men in the highest quintile had similar age-adjusted relative risk of stroke. In contrast, the age-adjusted relative risk for extreme quintiles of WHR was significantly higher. This relative risk was not substantially altered in a multivariate model including BMI, height, and other potential risk factors. The results suggest that abdominal obesity, but not elevated BMI, predict risk of stroke in men.

The role of abdominal obesity as a risk factor for ischemic stroke is still not completely known. Few studies have examined the relationship between abdominal obesity defined by WHR and stroke.

Increased visceral adiposity may be an independent risk factor of stroke rather than overall obesity. Markers of abdominal adiposity show a graded and significant association with risk of stroke/transient ischemic attack, independent of other vascular risk factors. Waist circumference can predict cerebrovascular events better than BMI. Abdominal obesity has been considered an independent, potent risk factor for ischemic stroke in all ethnic groups.

Visceral adipose tissue is associated with carotid intima–media thickness (c-IMT), plaque area, and total area (c-IMT area and plaque area combined) after adjusting for demographics, family history, smoking, and percentage body fat in men and women. In men, visceral adiposity is associated with c-IMT and total area after adjusting for insulin, glucose, homocysteine, blood pressure, and lipids. This association remained significantly associated with c-IMT after further adjustment for either waist circumference or WHR. Increased visceral adiposity is likely to represent an additional risk factor for carotid atherosclerosis in men.

Although increased visceral adiposity has been suggested to play a role in the development of ischemic stroke, the relationship between obesity and ischemic stroke remains less clear. The underlying mechanisms by which increased visceral adiposity can affect stroke risk, independent of established risk factors such as hypertension and diabetes, is not fully understood. It could be mediated by the pro-thrombotic (higher levels of plasminogen activator inhibitor-1 antigen and activity, fibrinogen, von Willebrand factor, and factor VII) and pro-inflammatory (increased levels of C-reactive protein and lymphokines) state in abdominal central obesity.

Prevention of obesity and weight reduction need greater emphasis in stroke prevention programs.

Key points

The evidence that obesity not complicated by hypertension, dyslipidemia, and diabetes is an independent risk factor for ischemic stroke is unclear and weak. By contrast, increased visceral adiposity appears to be a predictor of stroke, independent of BMI.

Adiposity-related risk factors for atherosclerosis

The pathophysiology of atherosclerosis in obesity is complex and is not completely understood. The combination of a cluster of anthropometric, hormonal, inflammatory, metabolic, hemodynamic, mechanical, pro-thrombotic, genetic, and environmental factors is probably necessary for the development and progression of atherosclerosis, coronary artery disease, and stroke in subjects with excess adiposity, as summarized in Figure 7.1.

Visceral adiposity

Visceral fat is an independent risk factor of coronary artery disease. The association of visceral adipose tissue with myocardial infarction is independent of traditional risk factors such as smoking, high-density-lipoprotein cholesterol, inflammatory markers, hypertension, and diabetes. The association between visceral adipose tissue and myocardial infarction is independent of the amount of total body fat. By contrast, subcutaneous and total fat mass appear not to be

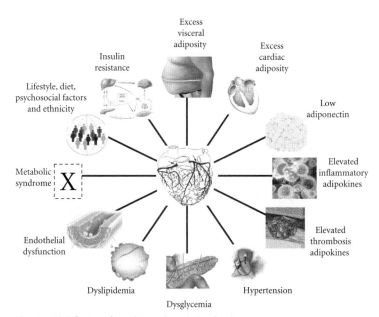

Fig. 7.1 Risk factors for atherosclerosis in obesity.

associated with atherosclerosis. Visceral fat deposition is significantly associated with calcified coronary plaques and with coronary artery calcium in young adults.

The relationship of visceral adipose tissue with myocardial infarction may vary with age and sex. Visceral fat has been reported to be an independent risk factor for myocardial infarction in women but not in men >70 years of age. Intra-abdominal visceral fat is associated with c-IMT, plaque area, and total area after adjusting for demographics, family history, smoking, and percentage body fat in men and women. Although the mechanisms for this causative role are still partially unclear, visceral adiposity seems to play an important role in determining coronary atherosclerosis. Visceral fat depots are the source of several bioactive molecules that, as a result of anatomical proximity, may influence and modulate the internal organs through endocrine and paracrine mechanisms.

Elevated secretion of pro-inflammatory and pro-thrombotic cytokines, increased portal release of free fatty acids, increased catecholamine-induced lipolysis, decreased activity of β_2-adrenoceptors, and decreased insulin-induced anti-lipolysis may contribute to the development of inflammation and insulin resistance and endothelial dysfunction, followed by atherogenesis.

Clinically, anthropometric surrogates of visceral adiposity are often used. Visceral fat is widely measured by the anthropometric markers of waist circumference and WHR. Although their accurateness is questionable, waist circumference and WHR are independent predictors of coronary artery disease and atherosclerosis.

Inflammation

Coronary artery disease and atherosclerotic plaque formation and pathological progression involve a complex inflammatory process. Obesity is associated with low-grade inflammation. Whether this is just an adaptive response to excess adiposity to maintain a normal oxygen supply or a chronic activation of the innate immune system is still unknown. Visceral adipose depots may react to chronic systemic or local inflammation, which may lead to coronary artery disease. The amount of adipose tissue and adipocyte size are both correlated with the number of macrophages, the direct source of inflammatory cytokines. However, both a direct and an indirect role of adipocytes in inflammation has been suggested. Adipose tissue may itself be responsible for the secretion of pro-inflammatory adipokines or, alternatively, may release factors that stimulate the production of inflammatory factors from other organs. These pro-inflammatory adipokines include tumor necrosis factor-α (TNF-α), interleukin-6 (IL-6), leptin, plasminogen activator inhibitor-1 (PAI-1), angiotensinogen, resistin, and C-reactive protein (CRP).

Clinically, obese patients generally present with elevated plasma CRP levels. Whether this is just an adaptive response to increased adiposity or represents a predictive role for CRP in coronary events in obese subjects is still unclear. Moreover, metabolically healthy but obese (MHO) subjects have a lower pro-atherogenic profile and inflammatory status than obese subjects with metabolic syndrome. Hence, the role of CRP as index of inflammation and as a prognostic marker of coronary artery disease in obese patients is controversial.

Endothelial dysfunction

Obesity is associated with altered arterial homeostasis and endothelial dysfunction. Endothelial dysfunction and inflammation interact significantly in obesity.

Endothelial dysfunction presents as inadequate vasodilatation and/or paradoxical vasoconstriction in coronary and peripheral arteries in response to stimuli that release nitric oxide (NO). A deficiency of endothelial-derived NO is believed to be the primary defect that links insulin resistance and endothelial dysfunction. NO deficiency results from decreased synthesis and/or release, in combination with exaggerated consumption in tissues by high levels of reactive oxygen and nitrogen species, which are produced by cellular disturbances in glucose and lipid metabolism. Endothelial dysfunction contributes to impaired insulin action, by altering the transcapillary passage of insulin to target tissues. Reduced expansion of the capillary network, with attenuation of microcirculatory blood flow to metabolically active tissues, contributes to the impairment of insulin-stimulated glucose and lipid metabolism.

Adipose tissue plays a major role in endothelial dysfunction through the secretion of pro-inflammatory cytokines, as described above.

CRP participates directly in the process of atherogenesis by modulating endothelial function. Elevated CRP levels induce overexpression of vascular cell adhesion molecule-1 (VCAM-1), intercellular adhesion molecule-1 (ICAM-1), selectins, and monocyte chemoattractant protein-1 (MCP-1) in cultured endothelial cells via increased secretion of endothelin-1 (ET-1) and IL-6. CRP attenuates basal and stimulated endothelial NO production by downregulating endothelial NO synthase mRNA and protein expression. CRP plays a direct role in obesity-related inflammation, but may also amplify the pro-inflammatory activity of other adipokines. Expression and activity of PAI-1, a pro-thrombotic cytokine frequently elevated in obese subjects, can be triggered by CRP in endothelial cells.

TNF-α, an inflammatory cytokine released at higher levels by obese patients, initiates and propagates atherosclerotic lesion formation. TNF-α may cause atherogenesis in part by inducing the expression of VCAM-1, ICAM-1, MCP-1, and E-selectin in aortic endothelial and vascular smooth muscle cells. TNF-α reduces NO bioavailability in endothelial cells and impairs endothelium-dependent vasodilatation, promoting endothelial dysfunction.

Adipocytes can directly induce endothelial dysfunction through leptin secretion. In fact, leptin upregulates ET-1, a potent vasoconstrictor, and endothelial NO synthase production in endothelial cells and promotes accumulation of reactive oxygen species. Leptin also stimulates the proliferation and migration of endothelial cells and vascular smooth muscle cells, as well as MCP-1 expression in aortic endothelial cells. Augmented angiotensinogen production by adipose tissue in obesity can induce endothelial dysfunction through the formation of free oxygen radicals from NO, thereby decreasing the availability of NO.

Insulin resistance

Insulin resistance can be defined as an inability or inadequate ability for insulin-stimulated glucose uptake by insulin-dependent tissues, as well as muscle and adipose tissue, and an inability or inadequate ability to suppress glucose production by the liver and kidney. Insulin resistance is associated with increased production of pro-inflammatory adipokines, as well as TNF-α and resistin, which can contribute to endothelial dysfunction and thereby to the development and progression of atherosclerosis.

A major contributor to the development of insulin resistance in obese subjects is an overabundance of circulating fatty acids. Once insulin resistance develops, the increased amount of lipolysis of stored triacylglycerol molecules in adipose tissue produces more fatty acids, which can further inhibit the anti-lipolytic effect of insulin, creating additional lipolysis. Upon reaching insulin-sensitive tissues, excessive fatty acids create insulin resistance by the added substrate availability and by modifying downstream signaling. As long as circulating free fatty acids increase hepatic glucose production and diminish inhibition of glucose production by insulin, lipogenesis will continue.

It is safer for the body to store triglycerides in small peripheral adipocytes. If the storage capacity of these adipocytes is exceeded, triglyceride accumulates in hepatocytes, skeletal myocytes, and visceral adipocytes. Additionally, a failure of adipocyte differentiation limits the pool of adipocytes available for energy storage, and excess triglyceride overflows to other sites, leading to insulin resistance. The abnormal triglyceride accumulation may lead to the development of hepatic and muscular resistance to insulin.

In obese subjects, particularly those with increased visceral fat, there is a strong association between inflammation, endothelial dysfunction, and insulin resistance/hyperinsulinemia. The combined effect of elevated inflammatory cytokines and insulin resistance/hyperinsulinemia can lead to endothelial injuries, and therefore increase the risk of development and progression of coronary artery disease in subjects with increased adiposity. The independent predictive role of fasting insulin and insulin resistance indices obtained from both fasting and non-fasting insulin has been described, but may be more modest than previously suspected.

Insulin resistance varies significantly among obese subjects. Obese subjects can be insulin-resistant, but they may also show preserved insulin sensitivity, as assessed by euglycemic hyperinsulinemic clamp studies. Moreover, obese subjects can be hyperinsulinemic and insulin-resistant, insulin resistant but without hyperinsulinemia, or hyperinsulinemic but without insulin resistance.

Clinically, fasting insulin and insulin sensitivity indices obtained from both fasting and post-prandial status, as well as the homeostasis model assessment of insulin resistance (HOMA-IR index), and values derived from an oral glucose tolerance test (OGTT) can be of help in providing information on insulin resistance in obese subjects.

Thrombosis

Obesity appears to be associated with thrombosis via several mechanisms. Obese patients, particularly those with predominant central visceral fat, have higher plasma concentrations of all pro-thrombotic factors (fibrinogen, von Willebrand factor, and factor VII) compared with non-obese subjects. Similarly, plasma concentrations of PAI-1 are higher in patients with visceral obesity compared with non-obese individuals. Obesity is characterized by higher plasma concentrations of anti-thrombotic factors, such as tissue plasminogen activator and protein C, compared with non-obese controls. The increase in these factors is likely to represent a protective response partly counteracting the increase in pro-thrombotic factors. Whether adipose tissue contributes directly or indirectly to plasma PAI-1 production is unclear.

Low adiponectin levels

Adiponectin is an adipocyte-derived plasma protein that accumulates in the injured artery and has potential anti-atherogenic and anti-inflammatory properties. Adiponectin exerts anti-atherogenic properties by suppressing the endothelial inflammatory response, inhibiting vascular smooth muscle proliferation, decreasing VCAM-1 mRNA expression, inhibiting the TNF-α-induced changes in monocyte adhesion molecule expression and in the endothelial inflammatory response, and suppressing the transformation of macrophages to foam cells.

Clinically, low plasma adiponectin levels have been observed in patients with obesity and coronary artery disease. Plasma adiponectin levels increase during weight reduction. Male patients with low plasma adiponectin levels (<4.0 µg/ml) may have a significant and independent increase in coronary artery disease prevalence.

Hypertension

Hypertension is a risk factor for coronary artery disease. Obesity is associated with elevated blood pressure. The risk of developing coronary artery disease in obese hypertensive subjects is significantly higher than in obese subjects with normal blood pressure. An increase in visceral adiposity is related to an increase in blood pressure and a cumulative risk of coronary artery disease. Obesity-related hypertension is discussed extensively in Chapter 8.

Dyslipidemia

Obesity is associated with an abnormal lipid profile and pattern. Increased visceral fat accumulation is a major risk factor for dyslipidemia. Obesity-related dyslipidemia plays a major role in the development of atherosclerosis and coronary artery disease in individuals with excess visceral adiposity. Obesity-related dyslipidemia is mainly characterized by increased triglyceride levels, reduced high-density lipoprotein (HDL) levels, and increased small, dense, low-density lipoprotein (LDL) particle number and composition. Other features of dyslipidemia related to abdominal adiposity include elevated levels of very-low-density lipoproteins (VLDLs), and reduced HDL_2, which is the large, buoyant, anti-atherogenic subspecies of total HDL. Apolipoprotein B (apoB) levels may be also elevated, reflecting an increase in the number of small, dense lipoprotein particles (VLDLs and LDLs).

The hypertriglyceridemia associated with visceral obesity and insulin resistance is related to the oversecretion of triglyceride-rich VLDL particles. An increased rate of hepatic free fatty acid uptake stimulates the secretion of apo B-100, leading to increased numbers of apo B-containing particles and possibly hypertriglyceridemia.

An increased number of small, dense LDL particles is an important feature of dyslipidemia in subjects with increased abdominal adiposity. When triglyceride levels are elevated, LDL particles become enriched in triglycerides and depleted of core cholesterol esters. Hepatic lipase then acts to hydrolyze these triglyceride-rich LDLs, forming smaller, denser LDL particles. Mechanistically, small, dense LDL particles enter the arterial wall more easily, bind to arterial wall proteoglycans more avidly, and are highly susceptible to oxidative modification, leading to macrophage uptake, all of which may contribute to increased atherogenesis.

Small, dense LDL particles are usually associated with a more atherogenic profile than large buoyant LDL particles. High levels of small LDL particles and increased inflammation are known to be associated with higher cardiovascular risk and, in particular, higher plasma triglyceride levels lower HDL cholesterol. The presence of small, dense cholesterol-depleted LDL particles is associated with an increased risk of myocardial infarction.

Obesity is associated with a higher number of small LDLs than non-obese subjects. However, MHO individuals have lower plasma concentrations of small LDLs and oxidized LDLs, suggesting that obesity alone is not necessarily associated with a higher number of small LDL particles. apoB and apoA1 are also considered atherogenic lipid particles. The apoB/apoA1 ratio has emerged as an independent reliable marker of hypercholesterolemia and a strong predictor of coronary artery disease.

Measurement of LDL cholesterol, triglyceride, and HDL levels is highly recommended in the clinical management of dyslipidemia in subjects with excess adiposity.

Dysglycemia

The association between elevated plasma glucose and coronary artery disease risk is a continuous variable. Obesity can be associated with a wide range of glucose abnormalities, usually termed dysglycemia. According to the World Health Organization and American Diabetes Association (WHO/ADA) criteria, dysglycemia includes impaired fasting glycemia (IFG), impaired glucose tolerance (IGT), and diabetes mellitus. IFG is defined as a glucose level between 110 and 125 mg/dl ($\geq$6.1 to <7 mmol/l) whereas IGT is defined as a 2-hour glucose level during a 75 g OGGT of 140–200 mg/dl (7.8 to <11 mmol/l).

Although the impact of frank diabetes on atherosclerosis and coronary artery disease independent of the presence of obesity is well known, the role of IFG and IGT is controversial. Hence, obese subjects may show no frank diabetes but may still have different levels of glycemia and high cardiovascular risk. In fact, IFG and IGT have been reported to provide a similar cardiovascular risk to overt diabetes. Non-diabetic levels of fasting and post-prandial hyperglycemia may be associated with an increased risk of cardiovascular disease. Elevated fasting plasma glucose and glycosylated hemoglobin (HbA1c) levels should be considered risk factors for coronary artery disease in non-diabetic obese subjects.

Measurement of fasting glucose and HbA1c levels are highly recommended in the clinical management of dysglycemia in subjects with excess adiposity. A 75 g OGTT can be also suggested to detect IGT in these subjects.

Epicardial adipose tissue

Although much of the attention has been focused on intra-abdominal fat, epicardial adipose tissue has been also considered as a visceral fat depot that may have a contributory role in the development of coronary artery disease because of its intimacy to the myocardium and coronary arteries and its biochemical properties.

Epicardial fat is the true visceral fat depot of the heart and is an extremely active organ that produces several bioactive adipokines. Because of its anatomical proximity to the heart and the absence of fascial boundaries, epicardial adipose tissue may interact locally and modulate the coronary arteries through paracrine or vasocrine secretion of anti- and pro-inflammatory adipokines. It is plausible that paracrine-released cytokines from periadventitial epicardial fat could traverse the coronary wall by diffusion from the outside in or could go directly into the vasa vasorum and downstream into the arterial wall. Local secretion of harmful, inflammation-producing cytokines from the epicardial fat could be predominant and could therefore down-regulate the production of protective and anti-inflammatory cytokines, as well as adiponectin, in severe and unstable coronary artery disease. It is reasonable to suggest that inflammatory signals from the epicardial fat could reciprocally be due to atherogenic inflammation in the underlying plaques. The regional ischemia could activate visceral adipose tissue oxidant-sensitive inflammatory signals in adjacent adipose stores. The presence of inflammatory cells in epicardial adipose tissue could also reflect the response to plaque rupture and could lead to amplification of vascular inflammation and plaque instability via apoptosis and neovascularization. On the other hand, synthesis and secretion of anti-inflammatory cytokines from the epicardial fat could be upregulated by improved local and systemic hemodynamic conditions. A dual role, both harmful and protective, for the epicardial adipose tissue has been suggested.

Clinically, epicardial fat thickness can easily be measured with a standard transthoracic echocardiogram.

Perivascular adipose tissue

Excess perivascular fat may play a role in atherosclerosis. Perivascular fat could potentially play a role in the morphological changes associated with an increase in vascular stiffness seen in obesity. Perivascular adipose tissue is likely to be a modifiable target, and a better understanding of its pathophysiological role may lead to the development of new strategies for the treatment of diseases associated with abnormal adiposity.

Ethnicity

As discussed previously, regional fat distribution can vary significantly among different ethnic groups. Given the key role of local body fat distribution in the development and progression of cardiovascular disease, the risk of coronary artery disease varies with ethnicity. In particular, South Asians show a higher cumulative cardiovascular risk when compared with Chinese and Caucasians. This finding seems to be related to the increased visceral adiposity that is frequently observed in South Asians.

Age

Aging by itself is a well-known major risk factor for coronary artery disease. Obese patients may be investigated for coronary artery disease at an earlier age than non-obese individuals, which may in part explain the recent lower prevalence of coronary artery disease overall in obese subjects.

Gender

Coronary artery disease is more common and its onset is earlier in men than in women. The incidence of atherosclerosis in women increases rapidly with the menopause. Gender-related regional fat distribution may play a role in the development of coronary artery disease among subjects with increased adiposity. Men tend to have more visceral and truncal abdominal obesity, whereas women usually have more subcutaneous peripheral fat accumulation. However, many obese women can present with the typical male obesity phenotype and therefore have similar cardiovascular risk to obese men.

Family history

Family history plays a significant role in coronary artery disease. Family history for obesity can act as an additional worsening factor for the development of coronary artery disease. However, the results are not univocal.

Physical activity

Individuals are considered physically active if they are involved in moderate (walking, cycling) or strenuous (jogging, football, vigorous swimming) exercise. A sedentary lifestyle and physical inactivity are emerging risk factors for both adult and childhood obesity. This type of lifestyle has a significant impact on the development of coronary artery disease.

Diet

Incorrect dietary habits including excess total calorie intake, excess intake of saturated fats, excess salt intake, and large portion sizes is a major modifiable risk factor for coronary artery disease. Three major dietary patterns and their impact on acute myocardial infarction risk have recently been considered by the INTERHEART study. An oriental diet was considered to have a high intake of tofu and soy and other sauces, a Western diet was considered to be high in fried foods, salty snacks, eggs, and meat, and a prudent diet was categorized as containing a high intake of fruit and vegetables. The prudent diet was clearly associated with a reduced risk of myocardial infarction, whilst the Western diet was weakly associated with an increased risk and the Oriental diet showed no significant relationship with myocardial infarction risk.

Smoking

Smoking increases the risk of coronary artery disease by 50% and the risk of an acute myocardial infarction by 40%, independent of obesity.

Alcohol

Excess alcohol intake is associated with increased risk of coronary artery disease, independent of obesity.

Psychosocial factors

Increased work and life stress can be a risk factor for acute myocardial infarction. A low socioeconomic status, a low level of education, and a low income can also be associated with increased obesity rates and can therefore lead to an increased coronary artery disease risk. Obese subjects may be more likely to become depressed, and depression is linked to increased atherosclerotic risk.

Metabolic syndrome

Metabolic syndrome is a long-term process, partially explained by the interaction of genetic and environmental factors, involved in the pathophysiology of atherosclerosis and coronary artery disease. The cluster of metabolic abnormalities that defines the presence of metabolic syndrome co-occurs in an individual more often than might be expected by chance. When these medical conditions are grouped together, they are associated with an increased risk of cardiovascular and coronary artery disease. Metabolic syndrome is a stronger predictor of coronary artery disease and total mortality than its individual components. Although several criteria have been proposed, two major definitions and criteria are currently used and accepted for the diagnosis of metabolic syndrome. These are summarized in Tables 7.1 and 7.2. Increased visceral fat accumulation, measured by waist circumference, is now considered a key factor in the development and progression of metabolic syndrome, although others consider insulin resistance and an abnormal lipid profile to be equally important as excess visceral adiposity. However, although insulin resistance is recognized as an important component of metabolic syndrome, its

Table 7.1 Definition of metabolic syndrome by the National Cholesterol Education Program, Adult Treatment Panel III, as at least three of the following five components

Central obesity	Waist circumference >102 cm in men and >88 cm in women
Elevated triglycerides	≥1.7 mmol/l (≥150 mg/dl)
Low HDL cholesterol	<1.03 mmol/l (<40 mg/dl) in men and <1.29 mmol/l (<50 mg/dl) in women
Raised blood pressure	Systolic BP ≥130 mmHg and/or diastolic BP ≥85 mmHg, or treatment of previously diagnosed hypertension
Impaired fasting glycemia	Fasting plasma glucose ≥6.1 mmol/l (≥110 mg/dl) or ≥5.6 mmol/l (≥100mg/dl)* or previously diagnosed type 2 diabetes

*The revised version recommended by the American Heart Association and the National Heart, Lung, and Blood Institute uses the lower cut-off value for impaired fasting glycemia. Reproduced from Grundy SM, Brewer Jr HB, Cleeman JI, Smith Jr SC, Lenfant C. (2004) Definition of metabolic syndrome: Report of the National Heart, Lung, and Blood Institute/ American Heart Association conference on scientific issues related to definition. *Circulation* 109:433–8.

Table 7.2 Definition of metabolic syndrome.

Central obesity, plus any two of the following four components	Ethnic-specific waist circumference criteria ≥94 cm in Europid men, ≥80 cm for Europid women
Elevated triglycerides	≥1.7 mmol/l (≥150 mg/dl) or specific treatment for this lipid abnormality
Low HDL cholesterol	<1.03 mmol/l (<40 mg/dl) in men, <1.29 mmol/l (<50 mg/dl) in women or specific treatment for this lipid abnormality
Raised blood pressure	Systolic blood pressure >130 mmHg and/or diastolic blood pressure >85 mmHg, or treatment of previously diagnosed hypertension
Impaired fasting glycemia	Fasting plasma glucose ≥5.6 mmol/l (100 mg/dl) or previously diagnosed type 2 diabetes

Source: International Diabetes Federation

measurement is not essential to the new definitions, whereas abdominal obesity plays a more critical role and is much easier to measure in clinical practice. Atherosclerosis is the primary pathological consequence of metabolic syndrome and develops through excess visceral adiposity, dysglycemia, the increase in LDL cholesterol and triglycerides, the decrease in HDL cholesterol, and the development of hypertension, inflammation, and endothelial dysfunction.

Metabolic syndrome comprises established risk factors for cardiovascular disease. Metabolic syndrome criteria are extremely helpful in identifying individuals who do not fit into the obesity categories, as defined by BMI, but who actually present with elevated risk of developing coronary artery disease and cardiovascular events. These patients, who are often asymptomatic, require an aggressive and adequate clinical approach and management to prevent major cardiac diseases. Additionally, some adiposity-related risk factors that are not presently included in metabolic syndrome definitions may confer an equally high cardiovascular risk and therefore require appropriate identification, assessment, and clinical management.

Adiposity-related cardiovascular risk markers

Waist circumference, triglycerides, HDL cholesterol, blood pressure, and fasting glycemia are considered the first-line clinically measurable cardiovascular risk markers in the management of subjects with excess adiposity.

Additional helpful cardiovascular risk markers in the management of obese subjects can also be considered. These second-line clinically measurable markers are CRP, LDL cholesterol, fasting insulin, the HOMA-IR index, the 75 g OGTT, HbA1c, and plasma adiponectin.

Ultrasound measurement of c-IMT and echocardiographic epicardial fat thickness can be considered third-line imaging markers of cardiovascular risk.

Although some indices are not yet fully established as predictive risk markers of cardiovascular events and atherosclerosis, the algorithm in Figure 7.2 has been suggested to improve clinical approach and management of obese patients.

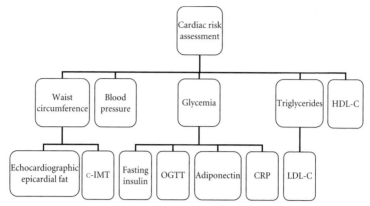

Fig. 7.2 Cardiovascular risk assessment in subjects with increased adiposity. HDL-C, High-density lipoprotein cholesterol; LDL-C, low-density lipoprotein cholesterol; c-IMT, carotid intima–media thickness; OGTT, oral glucose tolerance test; CRP, C-reactive protein.

Key points

Waist circumference, triglycerides, HDL cholesterol, blood pressure, and fasting glycemia should be routinely calculated in the clinical management of all subjects with excess adiposity and high risk of coronary artery disease.

Imaging assessment of coronary artery disease and atherosclerosis in obesity

Diagnosis of coronary artery disease and atherosclerosis can be challenging in the obese subjects. Imaging assessment of atherosclerosis in these patients can be difficult. Obesity can limit radiographic evaluation, and image quality may be lower because of the large body weight and amount of fat. Echocardiography is often the most affected. Nuclear imaging quality can be low in obese patients, and CT, magnetic resonance imaging (MRI), and X-ray tables may have weight limits that cannot be exceeded. The bore diameter of CT and MRI scanners can also be too small for the body girth of some patients.

Invasive coronary imaging

Coronary angiography

Coronary angiography remains the gold standard for diagnosing coronary artery disease. Cardiac catheterization using the radial artery or a femoral closure device is a safe method of evaluating coronary artery disease in morbidly obese patients. However, cardiac catheterization in morbidly obese patients can be difficult. The following technical problems that may occur, and which may limit the ability of these patients to undergo clinically indicated coronary angiography, include:

◆ difficult vascular access

◆ difficult radiographic penetration of the chest

◆ physical limitations of the table.

Non-invasive assessment of coronary artery disease may be indicated in morbidly obese patients who are unable to undergo coronary angiography.

Intravascular ultrasound

Intravascular ultrasound (IVUS) provides the ability to study vessel wall morphology *in vivo*, allowing accurate visualization of the details of vessel structure and tissue characterization. IVUS is usually performed at the same time as percutaneous coronary interventions. IVUS can be more accurate than arteriography in evaluating the deployment of stents in both peripheral and coronary arteries. IVUS can effectively assess coronary atherosclerotic morphology and function in obese patients who undergo cardiac or bariatric surgery interventions.

Non-invasive coronary and atherosclerosis imaging

Many non-invasive imaging techniques for coronary artery disease are available or under development, although there are few data on the application of these non-invasive procedures in obese subjects. However, non-invasive assessment of the coronary artery tree is desirable in obese subjects, particularly in those with co-morbidities and with a severe degree of obesity.

Nuclear medicine imaging

Nuclear imaging with radioactive isotopes of thallium (^{201}Tl) or technetium (^{99}Tc) can directly detect perfusion abnormalities in obese subjects.

Single-photon emission computed tomography and positron emission tomography Positron emission tomography (PET) is a nuclear imaging technique that uses short-half-life radionuclides incorporated into radiopharmaceuticals, allowing assessment of global and regional left ventricular wall motion and myocardial blood flow. Assessment of myocardial perfusion by single-photon-emission computed tomography (SPET) or PET appears to be valuable, even when coronary arteries are normal. Combined acquisitions by PET/computed tomography (CT) and SPET/CT hybrid systems can evaluate ventricular functions and myocardial metabolic state. Cardiac PET imaging has advanced from being primarily a research tool to being used as a practical, high-performance, clinical imaging method. Myocardial perfusion assessment by PET appears to be superior to SPECT in obese subjects.

Limitations of nuclear medicine in obese patients Nuclear imaging quality can be low in obese patients.^{99m}Tc (a metastable nuclear isomer of ^{99}Tc), which emits higher-energy photons than ^{201}Tl, is likely to provide higher-quality images in obese patients. Low image quality is especially problematic for myocardial perfusion SPECT in obese patients, as the small number of photons detected makes it difficult to know whether to attribute a detected drop in photons to a soft tissue attenuation artifact or to myocardial ischemia. The quality of PET images may also be lower in obese patients—image quality is degraded due to the high scatter in soft tissues and increased photon attenuation in a larger body mass. In addition, it may not be possible to give a large enough dose of isotope, as the maximum dose recommended for patient safety can often be well below the mCi/kg dose required for optimal image quality. In addition, extremely obese patients may not qualify for a nuclear stress test if their weight exceeds the weight-bearing limit of the nuclear imaging table (usually 140 kg). For such patients, stress echocardiography is the only feasible form of stress imaging.

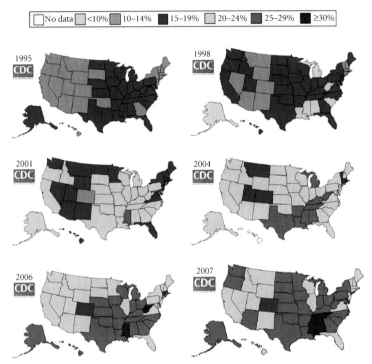

Plate 1 Obesity trends among US adults from 1995 to 2007 (see also Figure 2.4). Source: Centers for Disease Control (CDC) Behavioral Risk Factor Surveillance System (BRFSS) 2007.

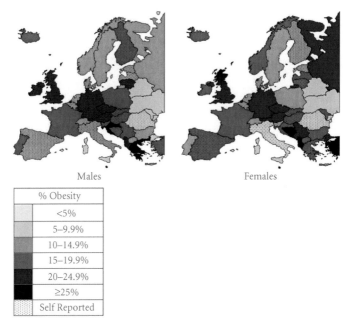

% Obesity
<5%
5–9.9%
10–14.9%
15–19.9%
20–24.9%
≥25%
Self Reported

Plate 2 Current prevalence of adult obesity in Europe (see also Figure 2.6). Sources and references are available from obesity@iotf.org. © International Obesity TaskForce, London – October 2007.

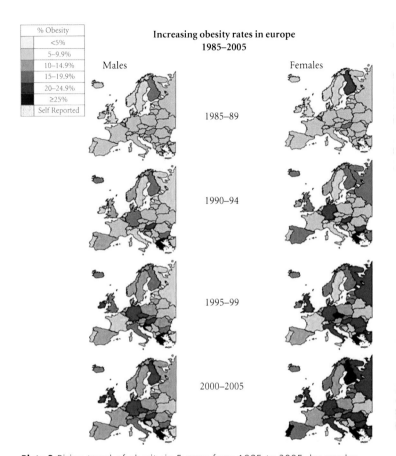

% Obesity	
<5%	
5–9.9%	
10–14.9%	
15–19.9%	
20–24.9%	
≥25%	
Self Reported	

Increasing obesity rates in europe
1985–2005

Males

Females

1985–89

1990–94

1995–99

2000–2005

Plate 3 Rising trend of obesity in Europe from 1985 to 2005, by gender (see also Figure 2.7). With the limited data available, prevalences are not age standardized and data from different years are not always directly comparable. The illustrations above are to give an impression of the changes that have taken place over the last 20 years. Self-reported surveys (illustrated with dots) may underestimate true prevalence. Sources and references are available from obesity@iotf.org. © International Obesity TaskForce, London – October 2007.

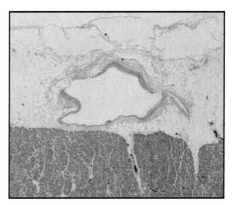

Plate 4 Close anatomical relationship between epicardial adipose tissue and the adjacent myocardium, showing the absence of a muscle fascia between them (see also Figure 4.2). Reproduced with permission from Iacobellis G, Corradi D & Sharma AM (2005) Epicardial adipose tissue: anatomical, biomolecular and clinical relationships with the heart. *Nat Clin Pract Cardiovasc Med* 2:536–43.

CT angiography

Although a CT scan can present technical problems in a severely obese patient, as discussed in Chapter 5, CT coronary angiography (CTCA) can provide complementary information on vascular structure and myocardial perfusion. In particular, multi-detector CT (MDCT) has been proposed as a non-invasive method of evaluating coronary anatomy. MDCT may be useful in excluding coronary disease in selected obese patients in whom a false-positive or inconclusive stress test result is suspected. A 64-slice CT scanner seems to provide accurate and precise imaging in severely obese patients. Dual-source CTCA provides high diagnostic accuracy to rule out coronary artery stenoses in patients with a high BMI.

Coronary artery calcification Coronary artery calcification detected by electron beam CT is a non-invasive index of coronary atherosclerosis. Coronary calcium assessment is of prognostic value in obese subjects with known coronary artery disease. CT-detected epicardial fat correlates with coronary artery calcification in subjects with increased visceral adiposity.

Cardiac MRI

Cardiac MRI clearly has the potential for assessing obese patients and has already emerged as a highly effective method of assessing ventricular function, myocardial mass, and myocardial viability in these subjects. Cardiac MRI angiography is a promising procedure because it is radiation-free, but its use in clinical practice is still under evaluation. Technical MRI limitations in severely obese patients have been described in Chapter 5.

Echocardiography

Although echocardiography can be difficult in obese patients, as discussed in Chapter 5, it can still be a helpful tool in assessing coronary flow. Non-invasive transthoracic Doppler echocardiography measurement of coronary flow velocity and the coronary flow velocity reserve of the left anterior descending coronary artery is feasible, even in a relatively obese patient. This methodology has the potential to provide useful physiological information of the functional significance of left anterior descending artery stenoses of intermediate severity.

c-IMT measurement

Carotid artery ultrasound can be performed with a 10 MHz linear-array transducer. c-IMT is calculated by measuring over a uniform length of 10 mm in the far wall of the right and left common carotid arteries within 2 cm proximal to the carotid bulb. The region with the thickest IMT, excluding areas with focal lesions, is measured.

Ultrasonographic measurement of c-IMT allows non-invasive and early detection of atherosclerotic changes and is used as a non-invasive end point for assessing the progression and regression of atherosclerosis. c-IMT is associated with coronary artery disease, increased visceral adiposity, and epicardial fat thickness. An increase in BMI is associated with an increase in c-IMT. The clinical use of ultrasonographic measurement of c-IMT in the management of obese subjects with increased cardiovascular risk is highly recommended.

Tests for inducible ischemia

A resting 12-lead electrocardiogram (ECG) is recommended in all obese subjects at risk of or with suspected coronary artery disease. The presence of T-wave inversion (2 mm) or Q waves suggests previous myocardial injury. ST–T depression and T-wave inversion during pain may be signs of myocardial ischemia. However, baseline electrocardiography may be not diagnostic, and can be influenced by excess adiposity, creating a false-positive diagnosis of inferior myocardial infarction, low voltage, and non-specific ST–T changes. If a resting ECG is not diagnostic, a stress test is suggested. Stress induction can be achieved by either physical exercise or infusion of pharmacological agents.

Exercise stress

Treadmill or bicycle exercises are performed most commonly. Exercise ECG is indicated to rule out coronary artery disease and vasospastic angina. It is also indicated for post-myocardial prognosis and for pre- and post-revascularization assessment. Criteria for a positive test are:

- planar or downward-sloping ST depression of at least 1 mm, 80 ms after the J point
- ST elevation

- increase in QRS voltage
- ventricular arrhythmias
- ischemia symptoms during exercise
- inability to increase heart rate.

Limitations of exercise stress ECG in obese patients

Conducting an exercise ECG may be difficult because of resting ECG abnormalities caused by obesity and difficulty in performing adequate exercise. Obese patients often have impaired exercise tolerance and thus are candidates for pharmacological stress in conjunction with an imaging technique.

Pharmacological stress imaging

Pharmacological stress imaging is the only feasible form of stress imaging in severely obese patients who are unable to exercise.

Stress echocardiography

Transthoracic echocardiography is the most frequently used imaging technique as it is less expensive and less invasive than other methods. After obtaining resting images, stress induction is performed and stress images are acquired. Echocardiography can visualize the transient regional wall motion abnormality induced by pharmacological stress. Dobutamine and dipyridamole stress echocardiography are the most common pharmacological stress tests. Dobutamine increases the heart rate and therefore increases myocardial contractility and cardiac demand. Transesophageal dobutamine stress echocardiography can be a good, safe alternative, although it is not widely used. Although obesity should be considered in the risk assessment of whether or not to perform dobutamine stress echocardiography, with proper precautions, transesophageal dobutamine stress echocardiography seems to be as safe in obese individuals as in non-obese. Dipyridamole induces a coronary supply–demand mismatch through alterations in the coronary blood supply.

Nuclear imaging stress

There are currently no robust data to support a role for stress imaging techniques in the risk stratification of obese patients. However, stress

^{99m}Tc-tetrofosmin SPECT myocardial perfusion imaging can be a useful tool for predicting cardiac and overall mortality in obese patients.

Management and treatment of atherosclerosis risk in obese subjects

Lifestyle changes

Lifestyle changes are highly recommended to reduce atherosclerosis risk in obese subjects, but they are often the most difficult to achieve. The key lifestyle changes required are quitting or avoiding smoking; weight loss, particularly when abdominal excess fat accumulation occurs; moderate but daily aerobic exercise for at least 30–45 minutes a day; correct dietary habits; and reduced alcohol intake, as summarized in Box 7.1. Detailed dietary and exercise guidelines are discussed in Chapter 13.

Box 7.1 Desirable lifestyle changes in subjects with increased adiposity

- Weight loss or avoidance of weight gain
- Moderate aerobic physical activity (at least 30–45 minutes a day)
- Correct dietary habits
- Stopping or avoiding smoking
- Reducing and avoiding excess alcohol intake.

Treatment of dyslipidemia in obese subjects

The treatment of dyslipidemia in obese subjects should focus on reducing the atherogenic lipid profile. LDL cholesterol is considered highly atherogenic and is therefore the primary target for the treatment of obesity-related dyslipidemia. Lowering small LDL particles and triglycerides and raising HDL levels are crucial secondary targets to reduce atherosclerotic risk. The apoB/apoA1 ratio has been also suggested recently as an independent and reliable atherogenic marker and as a strong predictor of myocardial infarction.

In obese subjects, reduction of the atherogenic lipid profile, and of an unfavorable lipid profile in general, including high levels of triglycerides and low levels of HDLs, can be achieved with lifestyle changes, substantial and sustained weight loss, and with lipid-lowering medications if lifestyle changes and weight loss strategies fail or are inadequate.

Therapeutic goals

Although treatments goals have been defined by the Adult Treatment Panel III (ATP III) for LDL cholesterol (Table 7.3), obesity is not listed among the risk factors that modify the treatment goals for LDL cholesterol in primary prevention. Hence, no specific recommendations for treatment goals for LDL cholesterol in primary prevention are available in obese subjects.

The following are suggested goals:

- Obese adults without coronary artery disease and LDL cholesterol concentrations range from 100–129 mg/dl should be encouraged to modify their lifestyle habits to minimize long-term risk

- In obese patients without coronary artery disease but with borderline high LDL cholesterol (130–159 mg/dl), sustained weight loss and lifestyle changes are needed both to lower LDL cholesterol and to minimize other risk factors

- If LDL cholesterol is high (160–189 mg/dl), clinical intervention with lipid-lowering drugs should be initiated in combination with weight loss and lifestyle changes

Table 7.3 Adult Treatment Panel III goals for LDL cholesterol levels

Category	LDL cholesterol (mg/dl)
Optimal	<100
Near-optimal	100–129
Borderline/high	130–159
High	160–189
Very high	>190

♦ If LDL cholesterol remains elevated despite therapeutic lifestyle changes, particularly when LDL cholesterol is >190 mg/dl, intensive lipid-lowering treatment should be considered.

These recommendations are summarized in Box 7.2.

The optimal treatment LDL cholesterol goal in secondary prevention, as well as in obese subjects with coronary artery disease, metabolic syndrome, diabetes, and hypertension, should be considered to be <2.5 mmol/l (100 mg/dl), as in non-obese subjects.

Lipid-lowering drugs

Lipid-lowering medications include inhibitors of 3-hydroxy-3-methylglutaryl-CoA reductase (statins), fibrates, selective cholesterol absorption inhibitors (ezetimibe), bile acid sequestrants (anion-exchange resins), and niacin (nicotinic acid).

Statins Statins are considered the first-choice lipid-lowering drugs. Statin treatment has been shown to improve the atherogenic lipid profile. Statins are extremely effective in lowering LDL cholesterol, and also in increasing HDL cholesterol and minimally decreasing triglycerides. Statins have been shown not only to reduce dyslipidemia, but also to reduce cardiovascular events and mortality, as well as the need for coronary artery by-pass grafting and coronary angioplasty. Statins can also induce regression of coronary atherosclerosis through a suggested beneficial effect on atherosclerotic lipid content and inflammation.

The most commonly used statins are simvastatin, atorvastatin, rosuvastatin, pravastatin, and fluvastatin. Doses can vary from 5 to

Box 7.2 Treatment goals for LDL cholesterol in obese subjects without coronary artery disease

♦ >190 mg/dl: weight loss + intensive LDL-lowering drugs
♦ 160–189 mg/dl: weight loss + LDL-lowering drugs
♦ 130–159 mg/dl: weight loss + lifestyle changes
♦ 100–129 mg/dl: lifestyle changes.

80 mg once daily. The starting dose depends on the initial LDL cholesterol value, and the presence of previous coronary artery disease and other obesity-related co-morbidities. The starting dose may also depend on the effectiveness of weight-loss strategies and lifestyle changes in lowering LDL cholesterol. A reduction in LDL cholesterol to <2.5 mmol/l (100 mg/dl) can be considered an optimal and desirable goal in the management of subjects with increased visceral adiposity and coronary artery disease. If the LDL cholesterol goal is not achieved, the statin dose can be increased gradually until the desired goal is achieved. An LDL cholesterol goal of <2.5 mmol/l (100 mg/dl) can usually be achieved with a high dose of a statin (40 or 80 mg).

Liver, muscle, and renal function should be monitored carefully in obese patients who are taking statins. Liver dysfunction occurs occasionally and is reversible. Rhabdomyolysis occurs rare, and severe muscle pain requires immediate cessation of therapy. Drug–drug interactions can commonly occur and deserve particular attention. However, combination lipid-lowering therapy is frequently needed to treat dyslipidemia when lifestyle changes are inadequate.

Fibrates Fibrates are used primarily for lowering triglyceride levels and increasing HDL cholesterol. They also minimally lower LDL cholesterol. The most commonly used fibrates are fenofibrate, gemfibrozil, bezafibrate, and ciprofibrate. Fibrates are very effective in reducing the atherogenic lipid profile, improving insulin sensitivity, lowering glucose levels, and raising adiponectin levels in obese subjects. Fibrates may increase the catabolism of all apoB-containing lipoproteins and reduce intra-hepatic triglyceride content in subjects with increased visceral adiposity. The mechanisms involved can be due to hepatic activation of peroxisome proliferator-activated receptors by fibrates, particularly fenofibrate at the dose of 200 mg once daily. However, fibrates are considered second-choice lipid-lowering drugs. They are mostly used in patients who are intolerant of statins or in subjects with prevalent hypertriglyceridemia and low HDL levels. The usual starting and recommended dose is gemfibrozil 600 mg twice daily and fenofibrate 160 mg once daily. The combination of statins with fibrates can be associated with a moderately higher risk of myopathy and rhabdomyolysis. Liver, muscle, and renal function parameters should be monitored carefully in obese patients who are taking fibrates in combination with statins. The risk is lower when a statin is used in combination with fenofibrate.

Ezetimibe Selective cholesterol absorption inhibitors, such as ezetimibe, can be used as monotherapy or in combination with statins in patients who are not reaching their treatment goals with statins or who are intolerant of statins and/or fibrates. The dose of ezetimibe is 10 mg once daily. The expected reduction in LDL cholesterol with ezetimibe used as a monotherapy is between 10 and 20%.

Bile acid sequestrants Bile acid sequestrants decrease total and LDL cholesterol, but tend to increase triglycerides. Although they are effective in treating hypercholesterolemia, the high rate of gastrointestinal side effects limit their use.

Niacin Niacin primarily increases HDL cholesterol, reduces triglycerides, and minimally reduces LDL. A new modified-release preparation (Niaspan) seems to have fewer gastrointestinal side effects and induces less facial flushing, factors that have limited use of the short-acting formulation.

Key points

Excess visceral adiposity is the major determining factor of dyslipidemia in obese subjects. Treatment of dyslipidemia in obese subjects should focus on reducing the atherogenic lipid profile. LDL cholesterol is considered the primary target. Different LDL goals can be identified. Therapeutic goals can be achieved with lifestyle changes, substantial and sustained weight loss, and lipid-lowering medications if lifestyle changes and weight-loss strategies fail or are inadequate. Statins are considered the first-choice lipid-lowering drugs for improving the atherogenic lipid profile and lowering LDL cholesterol.

Treatment of dysglycemia in obese subjects

Excess visceral adiposity is commonly associated with risk of developing overt diabetes or pre-diabetes, or dysglycemic conditions such as IGT and IFG that can lead to diabetes or may reverse to normoglycemic status.

Fasting blood glucose levels and a 2-hour blood glucose level measured using a 75 g OGTT are extremely important components in the assessment of an overweight or obese person, as patients with obesity (especially central obesity) are at high risk of pre-diabetes (IFG or IGT, or both) and type 2 diabetes (see Table 7.4).

Therapeutic goals

A reduction in both fasting and post-prandial blood glucose levels is desirable in obese subjects. Subjects with high visceral adiposity usually have elevated fasting glucose levels in the morning as a result of the increased overnight hepatic glycogenolysis and gluconeogenesis due to the high insulin resistance and excess visceral fat accumulation. HbA1c is generally accepted as a sensitive and reliable marker of overall glycemic control. The suggested goal in obese subjects is a HbA1c level of ≤7%.

Lifestyle changes

In obese subjects with IGT and IFG, it has been demonstrated that progression to diabetes can be prevented or delayed by lifestyle changes. Such changes are therefore highly recommended in obese subjects with pre-diabetes or with a family history of diabetes. Physical activity on a regular daily basis, correct dietary habits, and weight loss can prevent diabetes in susceptible obese populations.

Table 7.4 WHO classification of impaired fasting glycemia, impaired glucose tolerance, and diabetes mellitus

Glucose levels in venous plasma	Normal		Impaired fasting glycemia		Impaired glucose tolerance		Diabetes mellitus	
	Fasting	2 hours	Fasting	2 hours	Fasting	2 hours	Fasting	2 hours
mmol/l	<6.1	<7.8	≥6.1 and <7.0	<7.8	<7.0	≥7.8	≥7.0	≥11.1
mg/dl	<110	<140	≥110 and <126	<140	<126	≥140	≥126	≥200

Pharmacological treatment of obese subjects with dysglycemia

The addition of a selected pharmacological agent is suggested in overweight or obese adults with IGT and IFG or with risk factors for diabetes who are not attaining or are unable to maintain clinically relevant weight loss with dietary and exercise therapy, to improve glycemic control and reduce their risk of type 2 diabetes. There is evidence that diet and exercise combined with drug therapy are effective at preventing progression to diabetes in IGT subjects.

Metformin Metformin is a biguanide that decreases hepatic glucose output due to decreased hepatic gluconeogenesis and increased glycogenesis and lipogenesis, decreases intestinal absorption of glucose, and improves insulin sensitivity by increasing peripheral glucose uptake and utilization. Metformin also has a minimal weight-loss effect in overweight/obese subjects.

Metformin can be considered the first-choice pharmacological agent in overweight or obese adults with IGT and IFG or with risk factors for type 2 diabetes who are not attaining or who are unable to maintain optimal or adequate glucose control with dietary and exercise therapy. The starting dose can be 500 mg once daily at bed time and then increased gradually up to 2.5 g daily. Despite some gastrointestinal side effects, metformin is well tolerated by obese patients.

Renal insufficiency or a glomerular filtration rate lower than 60 ml/min are contraindications for metformin.

Anti-obesity medications Pharmacological treatment of obesity is discussed in Chapter 13. Contemporary anti-obesity drugs have been shown to impact positively on diabetes and pre-diabetes. Anti-obesity compound-induced weight loss has shown the potential to delay or reduce the development of dysglycemia and to significantly improve glucose control and HbA1c levels. Anti-obesity medications can be used safely with metformin, and the combination of metformin and anti-obesity agents can potentiate the anti-diabetic effect of weight loss.

Bariatric surgery

Bariatric surgery is an emerging and effective procedure for morbidly obese subjects with pre-diabetes. It is discussed in detail in Chapter 13.

Key points

Excess visceral adiposity is a risk factor for diabetes mellitus and pre-diabetes, such as IFG and IGT. A reduction in both fasting and post-prandial blood glucose levels is desirable in obese subjects. The optimal glycemic control goal is a HbA1c level of <7%. Lifestyle changes can prevent or delay the progression and development of dysglycemia. When pharmacological treatment is necessary to achieve the optimal glycemic goal, metformin is the first-choice drug in subjects who are obese but not yet diabetic.

Chapter 8

Obesity and hypertension

Definition of hypertension

The definition of hypertension and optimal blood pressure levels has recently been revised, as described in Table 8.1. The Seventh Report of the Joint National Committee on Prevention, Detection, Evaluation and Treatment of High Blood Pressure (JNC VII) indicates that blood pressure levels below 120 and 80 mmHg are now considered 'normal', whilst the previous categories of 'normal' and 'high–normal' have been combined to give the new classification of 'pre-hypertension' [systolic blood pressure (SBP) 120–139 mmHg or diastolic blood pressure (DBP) 80–89 mmHg].

The primary goal in the treatment of hypertension is to reduce morbidity and mortality by lowering blood pressure and by modifying other cardiovascular risk factors. The well-established relationship between blood pressure and the risk of cardiovascular disease is continuous, consistent, and independent of other risk factors. The higher the blood pressure, the greater the risk of heart attack, stroke, and kidney disease. In fact, for individuals aged 40–70 years, each incremental increase of 20 mmHg SBP or 10 mmHg DBP actually doubles the risk of cardiovascular disease across the entire range of blood pressures from 115/75 to 185/115 mmHg.

It is therefore recommended that clinicians should aim to normalize blood pressure and therefore in obese subjects it should also be reduced below 120/80 mmHg.

Excess body weight and hypertension

Obesity is a well-known risk and causal factor in the development of hypertension. Hypertension is about six times more frequent in obese than in normoweight subjects.

Table 8.1 Changes in the definition of hypertension and normal blood pressure

JNC VI	JNC VII	WG-ASH	Systolic BP (mmHg)		Diastolic BP (mmHg)
Optimal	Normal	Normal	<120	and	<80
	Pre-hypertension	or Hypertension	120–139	or	80–89
Normal		Stage 1	<130	and	<85
High–normal			130–139	or	85–89
Hypertension	Hypertension				
Stage 1	Stage 1	Stage 1 or	140–159	or	90–99
	Stage 2	Stage 2	≥160	or	≥100
Stage 2		Stage 3	160–179	or	100–109
Stage 3			≥180	or	≥110

JNC, Joint National Committee on Prevention, Detection, Evaluation, and Treatment of High Blood Pressure; WG-ASH, Writing Group of the American Society of Hypertension.

It is widely accepted that excess body weight is one of the strongest predictors of the development of hypertension. Many large epidemiological studies have demonstrated an association between body mass index (BMI) and blood pressure. The prevalence of elevated blood pressure defined as ≥140/90 mmHg increases progressively with increasing BMI among men and women, from 15% among individuals with a BMI <25 kg/m^2 to approximately 40% among those with a BMI ≥30 kg/m^2.

Even if daytime or work blood pressures are normal, 24-hour blood pressure recordings show that obese patients often have a 'non-dipping' pattern in which they lose the normal nocturnal decline in blood pressure.

Increased visceral adiposity and hypertension

Whilst it is true that excess body weight is associated with higher blood pressure, a body of evidences indicates that regional fat distribution, mainly visceral adiposity, plays an important role in the development of hypertension, rather than obesity per se.

Abdominal–truncal distribution of body fat is associated with increased blood pressure, independent of BMI. Subjects who present high abdominal–truncal visceral fat deposition are at higher risk of developing hypertension than subjects with more prevalent subcutaneous peripheral adiposity. Normoweight or overweight subjects with increased visceral fat should be monitored for blood pressure.

'Non-traditional' visceral adipose tissues, such as mediastinal and epicardial fat, have consistently been associated with hypertension.

Markers of abdominal–truncal adiposity, as well as waist circumference and waist-to-hip ratio, are better predictors of elevated blood pressure than BMI.

Key points

The prevalence of elevated blood pressure, defined as ≥140/90 mmHg, increases progressively with increasing BMI. However, increased visceral adiposity is more significantly associated with hypertension than overall obesity. Waist circumference is thus a better predictor of elevated blood pressure than BMI.

Pathophysiology of hypertension in obesity

The relationship between increased body weight and increased blood pressure is unquestionable, but it is complex and not completely understood. Several mechanisms can be evoked to explain the development of high blood pressure in obese individuals. The cause of hypertension in obesity is multi-factorial. Abnormal mechanical, metabolic, and biochemical variables interact and potentiate their impact on blood pressure in obese subjects. Possible causes and mechanisms of hypertension in obesity are summarized graphically in Figure 8.1.

Activation of the sympathetic nervous system (SNS) is a typical feature of obesity and seems to be a key mechanism in obesity-related hypertension, resulting in peripheral vasoconstriction, altered baroreflex activity, and increased arterial pressure.

The adipose tissue plays an active role in increasing the risk of developing hypertension in subjects with increased adiposity. Adipose tissue

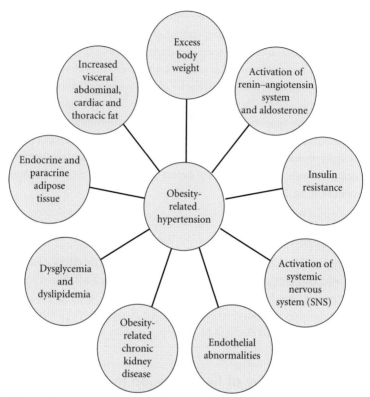

Fig. 8.1 The multi-factorial causes and mechanisms of hypertension in obesity.

functions as an endocrine and paracrine organ, and therefore produces hormones and cytokines that can directly or indirectly induce hypertension. These cytokines, called adipokines, can promote inflammation, thrombosis, lipid accumulation, and insulin resistance.

Obesity is commonly associated with insulin resistance, high plasma insulin levels, and low plasma adiponectin levels. Insulin resistance and hyperinsulinemia can increase sodium retention and volume expansion, and consequently increase pre-load. Insulin can also exert a direct growth factor effect on left ventricle (LV) chambers, LV mass, and the arterial wall.

Activation of the systemic and adipose tissue renin–angiotensin system (RAS) also has been implicated as a mechanism of obesity-related hypertension. Adipose tissue contains all the components of the RAS, which is upregulated in the presence of obesity. Upregulation of genes for angiotensinogen, renin, angiotensin-converting enzyme (ACE), and the angiotensin II type 1 (AT_1) receptor has been observed in obese hypertensive individuals.

Leptin, which is commonly elevated in people with obesity, is associated with increased heart rate, plasma renin activity, aldosterone levels, and angiotensinogen levels.

Endothelial abnormalities, such as decreased nitric oxide responsiveness, are also commonly observed in obesity, possibly due to increased production of endothelin-1, which induces vasoconstriction.

Obesity-related hypertension has recently been related to increased aldosterone plasma levels.

Obesity is also associated with increased renal SNS activity, which contributes to sodium retention and volume expansion. Obesity may cause glomerular hyperfiltration, increased urinary albumin loss and progressive loss of renal function caused by focal segmental glomerulosclerosis.

The large fat depots in significant obesity produce a low-resistance vascular circuit that may further increase cardiac output. The combination of these factors is proposed to produce a form of volume overload similar to that which occurs with regurgitant valvular heart disease, beriberi, or arterial–venous fistulas. Chronic volume overload or high output failure is classically thought to produce an eccentric form of cardiac hypertrophy with enlarged cardiac chambers but normal wall thickness.

Thus, there appears to be a slight predominance of concentric cardiac hypertrophy (increased wall thickness relative to chamber size) compared with an eccentric pattern of hypertrophy (chamber enlargement is more prominent than the increase in wall thickness). The pathophysiological mechanisms proposed to account for the presence of LV hypertrophy and the different patterns of LV geometry are discussed in Chapter 4.

Accurate measurement of blood pressure in obese subjects

The use of an appropriate cuff size for accurate blood pressure measurement is of crucial importance in obese patients. A longer and wider cuff is needed for adequate compression of the brachial artery in obese patients with a very large upper arm (Figure 8.2). Recommendations from the American Heart Association Council are as follows:

- For an arm circumference of 27–34 cm, the cuff should be 16 × 30 cm
- For an arm circumference of 35–44 cm, the cuff should be size: 16 × 36 cm
- For arm circumference of 45–52 cm, the cuff should be 16 × 42 cm ('adult thigh' size).

Twenty-four-hour blood pressure monitoring using a Holter monitor may be indicated in obese subjects with borderline or labile blood pressure values. Twenty-four-hour blood pressure monitoring may also be of help before and during treatment with sibutramine (see below).

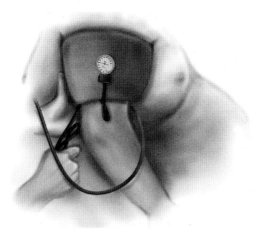

Fig. 8.2 Use of an appropriate cuff size for accurate blood pressure measurement in obese patients.

Clinical management of hypertension in obesity

Although obesity is recognized as a major cardiovascular risk factor, no specific guidelines for the treatment of hypertension or coronary artery disease have been proposed. However, in obese hypertensive subjects, it is reasonable to expect to achieve a blood pressure goal similar to that recommended for normoweight patients (<120/80 mmHg).

The first step in the management of elevated blood pressure in obese individuals should be weight reduction. Reducing body weight reduces blood pressure. Clinical trials have demonstrated that there is a diastolic reduction of 1 mmHg per kg of weight loss, and a 10 kg decrease in weight is associated with a decrease in systolic blood pressure of 5–20 mmHg. Weight loss also increases the response to antihypertensive treatment. However, because sustainable weight loss can be a difficult goal in clinical practice, a comprehensive approach involving both lifestyle modifications and pharmacological therapy is likely to be necessary in the majority of obese hypertensive patients.

Choice of anti-hypertensive drug in obese patients

Most obese patients with hypertension require two or more medications to achieve a desirable blood pressure level. When selecting therapy, physicians should consider not only the efficacy and safety of antihypertensive drugs, but also their potential effects on the cardiometabolic risk profile of the patient with both obesity and hypertension.

A possible therapeutic algorithm for the treatment of hypertension in obese patients is outlined in Figure 8.3. The advantages and effectiveness of the various classes of blood-pressure-lowering medications are presented briefly below.

First-choice medications

ACE inhibitors and ARBs

ACE inhibitors and AT_1 receptor blockers (ARBs) are widely used for the treatment of hypertension. Both classes of agent have been shown to reduce the cardiovascular morbidity and mortality significantly in patients with high cardiometabolic risk.

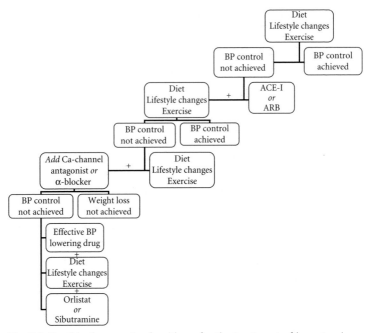

Fig. 8.3 Possible therapeutic algorithm for the treatment of hypertension in obese subjects. ACE-I: ACE-inhibitor; ARB: AT receptor blocker; BP: blood pressure.

Because of the previously described activation and upregulation of the RAS system in obesity, the use of RAS blocks and therefore of ACE inhibitors and ARBs may be specific, and provides benefits in the management of obese patients with hypertension.

In addition to their proven efficacy in lowering blood pressure, ACE inhibitors and ARBs have been shown to reduce proteinuria, sympathetic activity, oxidative stress, and LV mass; to improve endothelial and diastolic function; to increase levels of adiponectin; and to induce changes in adipocyte morphology and function. In fact, ACE inhibitors and ARBs have been suggested to facilitate the maturation from pre-adipocytes to mature adipocytes. Adipocytes are larger than pre-adipocytes, and have better insulin sensitivity and can lower lipolysis, which can result in a better metabolic profile.

ACE inhibitors and ARBs are generally well tolerated and may cause only minor side effects. However, recent trials clearly indicated that a combination of the ACE inhibitor ramipril and the ARB telmisartan was associated with more adverse events without an increase in benefit.

Key points

ACE inhibitors or ARBs in monotherapy can be considered the first-choice drug for treating hypertension in obese subjects. Additionally, because of the proven beneficial effect of ACE inhibitors and ARBs on several metabolic parameters and end-organ targets, these agents can be used in monotherapy for treating normotensive obese patients who are affected by type 2 diabetes mellitus, heart failure, or coronary artery disease. ACE inhibitors and ARBs may have a direct effect on adipocyte morphology and metabolism.

Second-choice medications

Calcium-channel blockers

Calcium-channel blockers are widely used in obese hypertensive patients. First-generation calcium-channel blockers are non-dihydropyridines, whereas the second generation are dihydropyridine L-type slow-channel blockers.

Calcium-channel blockers can promote natriuresis and reduce peripheral vascular resistance. Dihydropyridine calcium-channel blockers may be effective in obese patients with increased intravascular volume. However, the low peripheral vascular resistance that is commonly observed in obese hypertensive patients may limit their utility.

The non-dihydropyridine agent verapamil may be more effective in obese patients, as verapamil decreases heart rate, does not produce reflex activation, and may inhibit sympathetic activity. In addition, the combination of sibutramine and verapamil in obese hypertensive patients significantly reduces blood pressure and improves cardiometabolic profile without affecting heart rate.

α_1-Blockers

Doxazosin and other α_1-blockers are generally used in obese hypertensive patients. In addition to their efficacy in lowering blood pressure, these agents provide beneficial effects on the lipid profile and improve insulin sensitivity in dyslipidemic diabetic and non-diabetic obese hypertensive patients.

Third-choice medications

Thiazide diuretics

Thiazide diuretics are effective anti-hypertensive agents. However, they can have adverse effects on glucose metabolism through over-stimulation of SNS/RAS activity. Therefore, low-dose diuretic therapy is recommended in obese hypertensive patients. If adequate blood pressure control is not achieved, it is preferable to add an ACE inhibitor or an ARB agent, rather than increasing the diuretic dose.

β-Blockers

β-Blockers are effective in secondary prevention of coronary artery disease in obese hypertensive patients. β-Blockers also lower the risk of heart failure in obese patients. However, β-blockers tend to cause weight gain and may adversely affect lipid and glucose metabolism. β-Blockers may induce weight gain because of non-selective blockage of β_3-adrenoreceptors leading to a reduction in thermogenesis and calorie consumption.

Non-selective or β_1-selective β-blockers may decrease insulin sensitivity in hypertensive obese patients. Differences in the effects on glucose control among β-blockers can be observed and it has been suggest that carvedilol is more effective than metoprolol in obese hypertensive patients.

A combination of thiazide diuretics and β-blockers should be avoided in the clinical management of hypertension in obese patients.

Combined administration of sibutramine and anti-hypertensive drugs

As described in detail in Chapter 13, sibutramine is an effective and safe weight-loss drug. Because of its effect on blood pressure, some concerns have been raised about its use in hypertensive obese subjects. However, as also discussed in Chapter 13, its use has been positively reconsidered as safe and effective in these patients.

In hypertensive patients with well-controlled hypertension, a blood pressure decrease ($\leq$5 mmHg in SBP and $\leq$1 mmHg in DBP) is observed during treatment with sibutramine, even when the body weight remains unchanged. Concomitant use of other anti-hypertensive medication classes does not affect blood pressure reduction.

Sibutramine has not been found to induce or exacerbate hypertension when used at either of the two suggested daily doses (10 or 15 mg).

An anti-hypertensive combination therapy regimen with ACE inhibitors and calcium-channel blockers is more advantageous than a β-blocker/diuretic-based regimen in supporting the weight-reducing actions and concomitant metabolic changes induced by sibutramine in obese hypertensive patients. In fact, sibutramine-induced weight loss with long-term treatment may overcome the direct effects of this substance on resting blood pressure.

Key points

The first step in the management of increased blood pressure in obese individuals is weight reduction. ACE inhibitors and ARBs should be considered the first-choice drugs for treatment of hypertension in obese patients based on their demonstrated blood-pressure-lowering and metabolic effects. The management of obese hypertensive subjects may require combined administration of anti-obesity and anti-hypertensive drugs.

Chapter 9

Electrocardiography and arrhythmias in obesity

Electrocardiography in obese subjects

An electrocardiogram (ECG) is part of the routine assessment of subjects with increased adiposity and obesity. A resting 12-lead ECG is recommended. However, the ECG can be influenced by anthropometric changes and therefore may show abnormal results in obese subjects.

The major factors that can affect an ECG in obese individuals are summarized in Box 9.1.

Box 9.1 Confounding factors on electrocardiography in obese subjects

- Displacement of the heart by an elevated diaphragm in the supine position
- Increased cardiac workload with associated bi-ventricular hypertrophy
- Increased distance between the heart and the recording electrodes because of excess thoracic subcutaneous adipose tissue
- Potentially associated with chronic lung disease

Because of the complications of obesity and the accompanying adaptive morphological changes, obese subjects may present with pathological ECG or false-positive ECG alterations that may mimic pathological findings. Some typical ECG examples from metabolically healthy but obese (MHO) patients are shown in Figures 9.1–9.3.

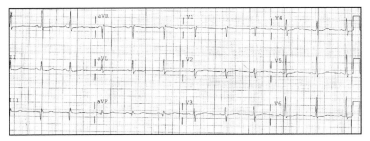

Fig. 9.1 Uncomplicated obese female, 57 years old: non-specific flattening of the lateral T wave.

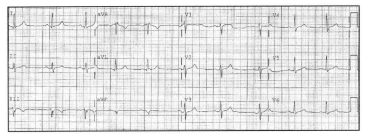

Fig. 9.2 Uncomplicated obese male, 34 years old: leftward axis, non-specific inferior T-wave abnormalities.

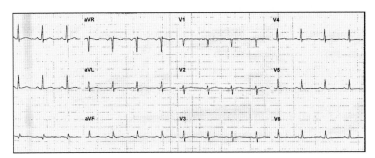

Fig. 9.3 Uncomplicated obese male, 67 years old: low voltage in the pre-cordial leads.

Heart rate can be raised as a result of the increased sympathetic tone commonly associated with obesity. Low QRS voltage, a leftward trend in the axis, and non-specific flattening of the T wave in the inferolateral leads, probably due to the horizontal displacement of the heart, are the most frequently observed ECG alterations in obese subjects. Obese individuals with increased abdominal adiposity may present false-positive criteria for inferior myocardial infarction. ECG in obese patients can show increased P-wave and QT dispersion, potential causes of atrial and ventricular arrhythmias. Obesity is also associated with an increased occurrence of abnormal, small, high-frequency ECG potentials (signal-averaged ECG or SAECG). Abnormal cardiac late potentials also occur among obese individuals without clinical cardiac disease symptoms, independent of hypertension or diabetes status. The most common ECG changes that are observed in obese subjects are summarized in Box 9.2.

Box 9.2 ECG changes observed in obese subjects

- Raised heart rate
- Prolonged PR interval
- Increased P-wave dispersion
- Prolonged QRS interval
- High or low QRS voltage
- Prolonged QT-corrected (QTc) interval
- Increased QT dispersion
- Increased SAECG (late potentials)
- ST–T abnormalities
- ST depression
- Left-axis deviation
- Flattening of the T wave (inferolateral leads)
- Left atrial abnormalities
- False-positive criteria for inferior myocardial infarction.

Electrocardiographic left ventricular hypertrophy in obese subjects

In obese subjects, the heart is shifted horizontally, presumably from the restricted diaphragmatic expansion caused by the increased abdominal adiposity. Hence, obesity may reduce the sensitivity of ECG voltage criteria for left ventricle hypertrophy (LVH) because of the attenuating effects of increased body mass on pre-cordial voltages. The most widely recognized ECG criteria for LVH are shown in Box 9.3.

Box 9.3 ECG criteria for LVH

- Sokolow–Lyon voltage criteria: $SV_1 + RV_{5/6} > 38$ mm
- Cornell voltage: R in a VL + S in $V_3 > 28$ mm in men and > 20 mm in women
- Cornell duration: > 2400 mm/msec
- Perugia score: ECG LVH is defined on the basis of one or more of the following being positive: (i) $SV_3 + RaVL > 2.4$ mV (men) or > 2.0 mV (women); (ii) LV strain; (iii) Romhilt–Estes score $= 5$

On the basis of several clinical and research studies, Cornell voltage criteria should be applied to assess ECG LVH in obese subjects because it seems to be less influenced by the presence of obesity.

Key points

In obese individuals, ECG LVH can be calculated using Cornell voltage criteria and is considered to present when the Cornell voltage is ≥ 20 mm in women or ≥ 28 mm in men.

Heart rate variability

Heart rate variability (HRV) is an index of the autonomic nervous system and measures the effect of the autonomous nervous system on the heart. HRV represents continuous fluctuations in heart rate.

HRV can be measured by R–R-interval variations on an ECG, or more accurately by power spectral analysis, which enables the identification of separate frequency components. The high-frequency component reflects parasympathetic activity, whereas the low-frequency component reflects mixed sympathetic and parasympathetic nervous system activity, although mainly sympathetic activity.

Obese individuals may have increased sympathetic activity, increased heart rate at rest, and reduced vagal activity. Obese subjects may have a decreased HRV and an abnormal cardiac autonomic nervous response to different stimuli.

Obesity and arrhythmias

Obese subjects have a higher risk of arrhythmias and sudden death than non-obese individuals, even in the absence of cardiac dysfunction, and independent of gender. Obese subjects may have normal heart beat, tachyarrhythmia, or bradyarrhythmia. The most common arrhythmias in obese individuals are atrial fibrillation and ventricular arrhythmias associated with a prolonged QT interval.

Investigations

Some investigations that can be of help in diagnosing and monitoring arrhythmias in obese patients are summarized in Box 9.4. A 12-lead ECG will certainly rule out regular or irregular rhythm and will

Box 9.4 Useful tests in obese patients with arrhythmias

+ 12-lead resting electrocardiogram
+ Blood tests (fT3, fT4, TSH, glucose, Ca^{2+}, Mg^+, K^+, cardiac enzymes)
+ 24 or 48 hour Holter ECG monitoring
+ Transthoracic echocardiogram (LV systole and diastole, LA dimensions)
+ Transesophageal echocardiogram (intracardiac thrombi).

provide information on the P wave, QRS complex and QT interval. A blood test is always indicated to evaluate thyroid hormones and glucose levels, electrolytes, and biochemical markers of myocardial injury. ECG monitoring for 24 or 48 hours using a Holter monitor may be indicated during anti-arrhythmic pharmacological treatments or to detect asymptomatic bradyarrhythmias. A transthoracic echocardiogram is indicated in obese patients with diastolic heart failure and atrial fibrillation for direct evaluation of LV systolic and diastolic function and left atrium (LA) dimensions, volume, and contractility. A transesophageal echocardiogram may be indicated to rule out the presence of thrombi in the LA in obese patients with atrial fibrillation.

Obesity and ventricular repolarization

QT-corrected (QTc) interval prolongation is a well-known risk factor for ventricular and fatal arrhythmias. Obesity is linked to changes in ventricular repolarization.

A positive correlation between QTc prolongation, QTc dispersion, and body mass index (BMI) has been described. Nevertheless, there is no significant difference on baseline QTc interval and QTc dispersion parameters between normoweight and uncomplicated MHO subjects. By contrast, a prolonged QTc interval can be observed in 30% of obese subjects with complications, particularly in those affected by diabetes and hypertension.

Obesity-related co-morbidities play a major role in affecting the ventricular repolarization rather than adiposity alone.

Specific instructions for the anaesthetic management of obese patients who undergo surgery may be necessary. Pharmacological agents that increase the sympathetic discharge or prolong the QT interval should be avoided.

Obesity and atrial fibrillation

Atrial fibrillation (AF) is the most common arrhythmia. It characterized by an ECG lacking any consistent P waves and a rapid, irregular ventricular rate.

Obesity is an important potential risk factor for AF. Obesity increases the risk of AF by 50%. The risk of developing AF increases progressively with increasing BMI, independent of age, sex, and hypertension. An association with BMI seems to be stronger for sustained AF than for transitory or intermittent AF. There is a progressive relationship between BMI and progression from paroxysmal to permanent AF.

The concomitant presence of diastolic dysfunction and AF could be early signs of the impaired systolic performance in morbidly obese subjects.

AF can be classified as:

◆ Paroxysmal if it is self-terminating within 7 days

◆ Persistent if it lasts more than 7 days

◆ Permanent if it does not terminate within 24 hours of cardioversion.

Clinical manifestations of AF

Many obese subjects have asymptomatic AF. However, the most common symptoms are palpitations, dyspnoea, and chest pain.

Possible mechanisms of obesity-related AF

Several mechanisms may explain the elevated incidence of AF among obese subjects and are summarized in detail in Box 9.5. Dilated LA, diastolic dysfunction, excess epicardial adiposity, and obstructive sleep apnea (OSA) have been suggested as the main potential determinants. Although the mechanism is still unclear, it is likely that a combined effect of these factors is necessary for the development of AF in obesity.

Investigations

ECG, blood tests, echocardiogram, and arterial blood gas analysis are recommended as first-line investigations in obese patients with new-onset AF (Box 9.6).

Treatment

Pharmacological treatment of AF in obese subjects does not differ substantially from that commonly applied to normoweight subjects.

Common therapeutic strategies have four main aims:

◆ Rate control alone

◆ Rhythm control

Box 9.5 Possible underlying causes of AF in obese subjects

◆ Atrial refractoriness heterogeneity may play a role in obesity-related AF

◆ LA dilatation, which is frequently observed in obese subjects, could be mechanistically involved in the pathogenesis of AF

◆ Impaired diastolic filling and abnormal LV relaxation, frequently observed in obese subjects, could lead to LA dilatation and subsequently AF

◆ Excess epicardial adipose tissue affects LA and diastolic function and may induce LA dilatation and therefore contribute to AF development

◆ OSA may play a role in AF development through hypoxemia, increased afterload, and pulmonary vasoconstriction. Nocturnal oxygen desaturation, which is an important pathophysiological consequence of OSA, is an independent risk factor for incident AF in individuals <65 years of age

◆ Increased oxidative stress or lipoapoptosis have been evoked as potential additional factors for AF in obese subjects

◆ Autonomic dysfunction and may also contribute to atrial electric instability in obese subjects.

◆ Controlling the patient's symptomatology

◆ Preventing thromboembolic complications.

However, the Atrial Fibrillation Follow-up Investigation of Rhythm Management trial has recently shown no survival benefits with a rhythm-control over rate-control strategy. A suggested therapeutic procedure for new-onset AF in obese subjects is summarized in Figure 9.4.

Rate control Rate control can be adequately achieved with pharmacological treatment. The first-line therapy is β-blockers or non-dihydropyridine calcium-channel antagonists (verapamil or diltiazem). The second-line therapy is digoxin.

Box 9.6 Useful tests in obese patients with new-onset AF

- 12-Lead resting electrocardiogram
- Blood tests (fT3, fT4, TSH, glucose, Ca^{2+}, Mg^{2+}, K^+, cardiac enzymes, drug levels)
- Arterial blood gas
- Transthoracic echocardiogram (LV systole and diastole, LA dimensions)
- Transesophageal echocardiogram (intracardiac thrombi)
- Chest X-ray.

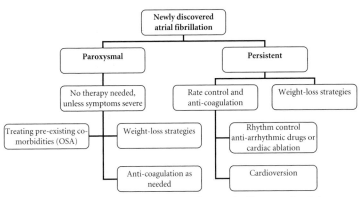

Fig. 9.4 Suggested therapeutic algorithm for newly discovered atrial fibrillation in obese subjects. Source: Fuster V, Rydén LE, Asinger RW, *et al.* (2001) ACC/AHA/ESC Guidelines for the Management of Patients With Atrial Fibrillation: Executive Summary A Report of the American College of Cardiology/American Heart Association Task Force on Practice Guidelines and the European Society of Cardiology Committee for Practice Guidelines and Policy Conferences (Committee to Develop Guidelines for the Management of Patients With Atrial Fibrillation). *Circulation* 104:2118–50.

Rhythm control When AF becomes persistent and symptoms are not diminished or improved with rate control alone, sinus rhythm restoration can be attempted.

Drugs Amiodarone is the most effective drug for rhythm control, although it can have toxic and non-cardiac side effects. Thyroid function and thyroid antibodies should be measured in all obese subjects before starting amiodarone. A pre-existing thyroid dysfunction may be precipitated or influenced by amiodarone. Other effective drugs for rhythm control alone are flecainide, propafenone, quinidine, disopyramide, and sotalol. However, their use in obese subjects should be limited as they may induce a long QT interval, observed in complicated obese individuals, and long QT-related ventricular arrhythmias. They are contraindicated in obese subjects with systolic dysfunction.

Catheter ablation Catheter ablation for AF is effective in obese patients. However, the recurrence of AF after ablation is higher in obese subjects. Additionally, obese patients may need to receive more than twice the effective radiation dose of normoweight patients during AF ablation procedures. Obesity needs to be considered in the risk/benefit ratio of AF ablation and should prompt further measures to reduce radiation exposure.

Pacemakers Pacemakers can be used for maintaining sinusal rhythm. Atrial pacing mode pacemakers (AAI or DDD) are mandatory because they reduce the AF burden.

Treating of pre-existing co-morbidities When OSA and AF coexist, treatment for OSA may improve and assist in the management of AF.

Anti-coagulant therapy Anti-coagulation in AF is requested for thromboembolism prevention. However, safe and effective use of anti-coagulant therapy may require a consideration of obesity. Obese patients may present potential problems for decisions regarding weight-based dosing of several anti-coagulants. Concerns have been raised about the appropriate dose of low-molecular-weight heparin needed to provide an anti-coagulant response in obese patients.

Anti-platelet-aggregation therapy Obese insulin-resistant subjects may have a blunted response to the platelet-inhibitory effect of aspirin. It is possible that insulin-resistant obese subjects might benefit from aspirin at a higher dose than insulin-sensitive subjects, or from therapies inhibiting platelet aggregation by blocking thromboxane-independent pathways or thromboxane receptors.

Obesity-related atrial fibrillation and cardiac surgery

Obesity may contribute to new-onset AF after cardiac surgery. Post-operative AF usually occurs within 5 days of open-heart surgery, with a peak incidence on the second day. Unless contraindicated, treatment with an oral β-blocker to prevent post-operative AF is recommended for obese patients undergoing cardiac surgery. Pre-operative administration of amiodarone may reduce the incidence of AF in obese patients who undergo cardiac surgery and represents an appropriate prophylactic therapy for obese subjects at high risk of post-operative AF.

Key points

Obese subjects, particularly those with metabolic complications and OSA, are at high risk of developing AF. ECG, blood tests, echocardiogram, and arterial blood gas analysis are recommended as first-line investigations in obese patients with newly discovered AF. Rate control and anti-coagulation treatment are effective in treating persistent AF.

Effect of weight loss on electrocardiogram parameters

Weight loss can induce significant amelioration in some ECG parameters. Weight loss may induce a rightward shift of the QRS axis. In addition, autonomic abnormalities improve after weight loss. Diet and surgically induced substantial weight loss in obese subjects is associated with a decrease in P-wave duration and dispersion. Substantial weight loss in obese subjects is accompanied by a significant shortening of the prolonged QT interval and decreased QTc dispersion. The degree of QTc dispersion reduction is associated with the amount of weight loss. Surgically induced weight loss is associated with a significant decrease in the heterogeneity of ventricular repolarization, as well as a reduction in spatial and transmural dispersion of repolarization. These weight-loss-induced ECG changes may explain the reduction in the risk of potentially fatal and non-fatal arrhythmias in morbidly obese subjects.

> **Key point**
>
> Obesity is associated with a wide variety of ECG changes, many of which can be corrected by weight loss.

Chapter 10

Obesity and heart failure

Risk of heart failure

Heart failure can be defined as when the heart fails to pump blood at a rate commensurate with metabolic requirements. Previous cardiac abnormalities or predisposing cardiovascular diseases that negatively affect heart morphology and function are necessary for the development of heart failure. The prevalence of heart failure is increasing, and novel risk factors have been identified and traditional ones have been revisited.

Obesity has traditionally been considered a risk factor for heart failure. However, the relationship between obesity and heart failure is complex and is not completely understood. Obesity, defined on the basis of body mass index (BMI), has been reported to double the risk of developing heart failure. In fact, the Framingham Heart Study showed that, after correction for other risk factors, for every one-point increase in BMI, the increase in risk of developing cardiac failure was 5% in men and 7% in women. This increased risk was evident in both sexes and was not limited to subjects with extreme obesity.

However, increased BMI and therefore obesity is also a risk factor for hypertension, coronary artery disease, diabetes mellitus, and dyslipidemia, all of which can independently increase the risk of heart failure. A smaller effect of BMI on the risk of heart failure in subjects with hypertension has been observed. This finding indicates that obesity is likely to provide only a small contribution to the risk of heart failure in the presence of these other major risk factors.

Thus, although obesity complicated by major cardiometabolic diseases can be a risk factor for heart failure, the role of obesity alone in causing heart failure seems to be weak or at least uncertain.

Possible pathophysiology of heart failure

Hypertension, diabetes, and coronary artery diseases play the major causative role in the development of heart failure in morbidly obese subjects. Complicated obesity predisposes to clinical heart failure because of the presence of one or more of these co-morbidities and their intrinsic pathophysiological mechanisms.

Uncomplicated obesity is usually associated with appropriate left ventricular (LV) remodeling, diastolic dysfunction, and normal or hyperdynamic systolic function. Hence, obesity by itself seems unlikely to predispose to heart failure.

It is therefore difficult to identify the pathophysiological mechanisms that can induce heart failure independent of obesity-related complications. Mechanical, hemodynamic, and hormonal factors have been suggested to explain heart failure in obese subjects.

Obesity is associated with an expanded intravascular volume, which can result in increased pre-load and cardiopulmonary volume. Obesity may contribute to heart failure by additional mechanisms, including adipokine release, neurohormonal activation and increased oxidative stress, infiltration of myocytes with free fatty acids, and B-type natriuretic peptide depletion. The natriuretic peptide system and adiposity seem to be linked—natriuretic peptide levels are reduced in obese patients with heart failure.

Insulin resistance is likely to account for some, but not all, of this association. The mechanisms by which insulin resistance and obesity promote heart failure risk remain uncertain. Proposed mechanisms include a systemic inflammatory state with increased concentrations of circulating inflammatory mediators such as C-reactive protein, plasminogen activator inhibitor-1, tumor necrosis factor-α (TNF-α), interleukin-6 (IL-6), angiotensinogen, vascular endothelial growth factor, and serum amyloid A3. Increased circulating concentrations of tumor necrosis factor-α, interleukin-6, and C-reactive protein have been associated with increased incidence of heart failure. Elevated circulating levels of resistin have also recently been associated with increased risk of new-onset heart failure. The association of resistin with heart failure persists after adjustment for established heart failure risk factors, obesity, markers of insulin resistance and inflammation, and concentrations of B-type natriuretic peptide, and after exclusion of prevalent and incident coronary heart disease. The role of adiponectin in the development of heart failure remains uncertain.

Taken together, these mechanical, hemodynamic, and hormonal factors may cumulatively increase the risk of developing heart failure, although the risk is more closely linked to the major cardiometabolic diseases associated with morbid obesity.

Key points

The relationship of obesity and heart failure is complex and remains unclear. An increase in BMI increases the risk of developing heart failure. However, morbidly obese subjects are more likely to develop heart failure as a result of the complications of obesity, rather than the increased adiposity itself. Mechanical, hemodynamic, and hormonal factors may contribute to increase the risk of heart failure in morbidly obese subjects.

Prognosis and outcome of heart failure

Whilst it is true that obesity is a risk factor for heart failure, the prevalence of heart failure among obese subjects has also been considered from a different perspective. Evidence-based medical studies have indicated recently that the relationship between heart failure and obesity should be reconsidered.

Recent data suggest a protective effect of obesity on heart failure outcomes and prognosis, which has been called the 'obesity paradox'. In fact, subjects with established heart failure who are obese have a paradoxically more favorable clinical prognosis than normoweight subjects with heart failure. In different hospitalized patients with heart failure, a higher BMI was unexpectedly associated with a lower hospital mortality risk. Overweight and obese subjects are associated with lower all-cause mortality when compared with normoweight individuals, whereas underweight and low–normal weight patients with stable congestive heart failure are associated with higher cardiovascular mortality. Even after adjustment for traditional cardiovascular risk factors, obesity and overweight are still associated with a lower risk of mortality for heart failure.

These findings indicate that obesity is not automatically associated with increased mortality for acute heart failure and may paradoxically confer a more favorable prognosis. However, the paradoxical relationship between obesity and adverse outcomes in heart failure is complex and is not completely understood.

The following explanations for the protective effect of obesity on heart failure outcomes have been proposed:

- Obesity may improve heart failure survival because it counteracts the adverse effect of cachexia, commonly observed in subjects with heart failure

- Obese patients may present earlier or have co-morbidities that are more readily recognized and more aggressively treated

- Obese patients with heart failure are usually younger than normoweight subjects presenting with heart failure

- Increased subcutaneous fat could provide a more favorable effect than visceral fat deposition; therefore, obesity should be defined based regional fat distribution markers rather than on BMI

- The overall number of metabolically healthy but obese (MHO) subjects may be underestimated, which may explain the low prevalence of heart failure and its better outcome in obese subjects

- Cytokine production and the neuroendocrine profiles of obese patients may play a role in modulating heart failure progression

- Preserved baseline systolic function may explain the increased survival rate of obese patients among individuals with congestive heart failure. Hence, obese patients who present with previous systolic dysfunction may be at increased risk of mortality for heart failure.

Key points

Obesity is associated with a better prognosis and lower cardiovascular mortality rates in patients with heart failure. Obesity may provide a protective effect on the progression and outcome of heart failure. This is known as the 'obesity paradox'. The reason for this effect is currently unknown.

Diagnosis of heart failure

Clinical diagnosis of heart failure in obese subjects does not differ substantially from that in normoweight subjects.

The major criteria of heart failure include paroxysmal nocturnal dyspnea, orthopnea, jugular venous distension, hepatojugular reflux, pulmonary crackles (rales), radiographic evidence of cardiomegaly, acute pulmonary edema, third heart sound, central venous pressure >16 cm of water, and weight loss >4.5 kg during the first 5 days of treatment for suspected heart failure.

The minor criteria of heart failure include bilateral ankle edema, nocturnal cough, dyspnea on ordinary exertion, hepatomegaly, pleural effusion, and a heart rate >120 beats/min.

Diagnostic use of B-type natriuretic peptide

In addition to these well-established clinical criteria, recent evidence suggests that the use of B-type natriuretic peptide (BNP) for early diagnosis of heart failure is helpful in asymptomatic or pauci-symptomatic morbidly obese subjects. In fact, reduced levels of circulating natriuretic peptides may be related to earlier expression of heart failure in the presence of obesity.

BNP is a 32 amino acid protein synthesized by the myocardium. BNP can be helpful in making a diagnosis of heart failure, even when standard clinical assessment is not informative. Both the N-terminal fragment of BNP (NT-proBNP) and BNP itself can be measured in the peripheral blood of patients with congestive heart failure. A cut-off point for BNP of ≥100 pg/ml has been suggested for the diagnosis of heart failure. However, there is an inverse relation between BNP levels and BMI. In fact, obesity is associated with lower BNP levels in healthy individuals and patients with chronic congestive heart failure. Both NT-proBNP and BNP levels decrease with increasing BMI.

BMI influences the selection of cut-off points for BNP in diagnosing acute heart failure. A lower cut-off point (BNP ≥54 pg/ml) should be used in severely obese patients to preserve sensitivity. A higher cut-off point in lean patients (BNP ≥170 pg/ml) can be used to increase specificity.

Key points

Assessment of BNP levels can be helpful in making a diagnosis of heart failure. BNP is lower in obese patients. A cut-off point for BNP of ≥54 pg/ml for diagnosing acute heart failure should be used in severely obese patients.

Heart failure management

Pharmacological treatment of congestive heart failure in obese subjects does not differ substantially from that in normoweight subjects. Optimal medical treatment, lifestyle changes, and appropriate weight loss should be part of the management of heart failure in obese subjects (Figure 10.1).

Weight loss in heart failure management

Correct and appropriate dietary habits should be considered for both prevention and management of heart failure in obese individuals. Appropriate weight loss in heart-failure patients with morbid obesity has been associated with improvements in systolic and diastolic function and heart failure classification. In order to prevent cachexia, a

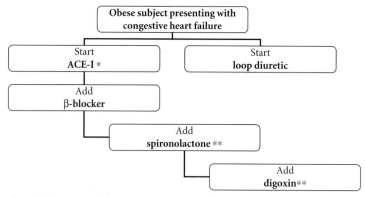

Fig. 10.1 Suggested therapeutic algorithm for congestive heart failure in obese subjects. *, ACE-I, ACE inhibitors; consider ARBs if ACE inhibitors are not tolerated. **, Add spironolactone and/or digoxin if the patient is still symptomatic.

tailored dietetic program may improve clinical and instrumental parameters in patients with heart failure. Weight loss may lead to an improved functional status, and to a reduction in LV remodeling and an increase in the ejection fraction. A team approach with cardiologists, endocrinologist, and nutritionists is desirable for optimal dietary strategies in patients with acute and chronic heart failure.

Key point

The management of heart failure in obese subjects should include optimal medical treatment and tailored weight-loss strategies.

Chapter 11

Obesity and peripheral venous diseases

Obesity and chronic venous disease

Obesity is often associated with venous insufficiency and chronic venous disease. Severely obese subjects frequently present with pedal edema, partly due to elevated ventricular filling pressure. Obese subjects with decreased mobility can also have high volume lymphatic overload and increased intravascular volume. These factors may reduce the pumping function of calf and leg muscles and therefore result in reflux of blood in the leg veins attributable to venous valvular incompetence. The reflux pattern and BMI are clinically correlated. Severe obesity increases the risk of severe and sustained lower extremity venous stasis disease, pre-tibial ulceration, and cellulitis.

Obesity and venous thromboembolism

Venous thromboembolism is a common disease with an incidence of 1.4 per 1000 person years.

Although there is some conflicting evidence, obesity is a common risk factor for venous thromboembolism. Obesity is a major risk factor for venous thromboembolic disease in both men and women. Obesity increases the risk of deep vein thrombosis (DVT), including after surgery. Obesity can be associated with an increased risk of pulmonary embolism, although this is still unclear. Whether the impact of excess body weight by itself or obesity-related complications is more important for the risk of venous thrombosis and thromboembolism remains unclear.

The risk of venous thromboembolism attributable to obesity has been assessed in both retrospective and prospective studies. In a National Hospital Discharge Survey, the relative increased risk of DVT in obese patients compared with non-obese patients was found to be 2.50. Obese female subjects have a greater relative risk of DVT than obese males (2.75 versus 2.02). Obesity has the greatest impact on both men and women of less than 40 years. In a retrospective, population-based US study, a 10-point increase in BMI was found to increase the risk of recurrent venous thromboembolism by 24%. In another retrospective analysis, increased BMI was associated with a higher probability of recurrent venous thromboembolism among young women. A non-significant 1.9-fold increase in the risk of recurrence was also seen in European patients with a BMI >30 kg/m^2 compared with those with a lower BMI.

Prospective studies have shown that excess body weight is a risk factor for recurrent venous thromboembolism. In a Nurses' Health study, higher BMI was found to be an independent risk factor for pulmonary embolism. In a retrospective hospital discharge set, obese men and women had a two- and threefold increased risk of venous thromboembolism, respectively. Excess body weight is also a risk factor for venous thromboembolism among medical and surgical patients. Additionally, there is a linear correlation between the risk of recurrence with increasing body weight in patients with a first unprovoked venous thromboembolism. The effect of excess body weight on risk of recurrence seems to be independent of age and sex. Risk of recurrence is 30% higher among overweight patients and 60% higher among obese patients when compared with patients of normal weight. Obesity confers the highest risk, resulting in an almost twofold increased risk of recurrence among patients with a BMI of 40 kg/m^2. In several reports, obesity has been found to be a risk factor for venous thromboembolism in the post-operative phase, among women using oral contraceptives, in the antepartum and post-partum periods, and among hospitalized patients.

Few studies have shown that obesity is a risk factor for pulmonary embolism in the general population, and this association was shown only among women. A National Hospital Discharge Survey showed that the relative risk of pulmonary embolism was 2.21 in obese women compared with normoweight women.

Mechanisms of venous thrombosis in obese subjects

The mechanisms by which excess body weight is associated with venous thrombosis are not completely understood. Obesity is thought to predispose to venous stasis, which is a trigger for DVT. Excess body weight has also been related to various alterations in the coagulation system, including impaired fibrinolytic activity and elevated plasma concentrations of clotting factors. D-dimer, fibrinogen, factor VIII, and factor IX increase significantly with an increase in BMI. In addition, the increased chronic low-grade inflammatory status commonly observed in obese subjects may contribute to the hypercoagulable state and thrombus formation. Central and abdominal obesity is associated with changes in hemostasis. Central obesity may increase the risk of a venous thromboembolism as a result of changes in haemostasis and possibly in the fibrinolytic system.

Increased visceral adiposity is also considered an independent risk factor for venous thromboembolism. Waist circumference has been reported to be more predictive of a venous thromboembolism than BMI. Waist circumference is independently related to the incidence of venous thromboembolism. Men with a larger waist circumference appear to have a fourfold higher risk of venous thromboembolism than men with a lower waist circumference.

Diagnosis of deep vein thrombosis

Diagnosis of venous thrombosis in severely obese patients can be challenging. These patients are difficult to examine physically and often have subtle first signs. Minimally symptomatic deep venous thrombi can be underestimated and often progress to fatal pulmonary emboli.

Diagnosis of DVT should be made by a combination of clinical signs and symptoms, and by the finding of at least one of the following criteria on venography or on color duplex sonography.

Venography diagnostic criteria of DVT are one of the following:

- ◆ A constant filling defect seen on two views
- ◆ An abrupt discontinuation of the contrast-filled vessel at a constant level of the vein
- ◆ The absence of filling in the entire deep vein system (without a compression) with or without venous flow through collateral veins.

Color duplex sonography diagnostic criteria of DVT are one of the following:

♦ Visualization of an intraluminal thrombus in a deep vein

♦ Incomplete or absent compressibility.

Recurrent non-fatal DVT is defined as a new non-compressible vein segment, an increase in the vein diameter of >4 mm compared with the last available measurement on venous ultrasonography, or a new intraluminal filling defect on venography.

Diagnosis of pulmonary embolism

The diagnosis of pulmonary embolism is confirmed either by a positive finding on a ventilation/perfusion scan, according to the criteria of the Prospective Investigation of Pulmonary Embolism Diagnosis, or by spiral computed tomography (CT) revealing one or more low-attenuation areas that partly or completely fill the lumen of an opacified vessel.

Recurrent non-fatal pulmonary embolism is defined as a new ventilation/perfusion mismatch on a lung scan or a new intraluminal filling defect on spiral CT of the chest.

Clinical management and prevention strategies

Preventing venous thromboembolism is unquestionably essential. Given the fact that excess body weight confers an increased risk of first and recurrent venous thrombosis and venous thromboembolism events, management of these patients is important.

Low-molecular-weight heparin (LMWHs) preferentially inactivates factor Xa. Hence, anti-factor Xa monitoring may be useful in obese patients who are on LMWH, although the results are controversial. It has been recommended that obese patients should have periodic monitoring of anti-factor Xa activity during treatment with LMWH. However, this does not appear to be necessary in patients with a body weight lower than 190 kg. In patients who weigh less than 190 kg, the available data indicate that the response to weight-based LMWH dosing is not affected. It is important that LMWH dosing is based on actual body weight. If the patient weighs more than 190 kg and anti-factor Xa monitoring is available, LMWH therapy may be based on actual body weight with dosage adjustments based on anti-factor Xa levels. If anti-factor Xa monitoring is not available for patients weighing more than 190 kg, LMWH therapy should be dosed according to actual body weight, and, if bleeding occurs, the dosage should be reduced.

The optimal duration of anti-coagulation treatment for a first episode of venous thromboembolism is uncertain. Predictive markers of venous thromboembolism recurrence may identify low-risk patients who are less likely to benefit from prolonged anti-coagulation. It has been reported that, in patients who have completed at least 3 months of anti-coagulation treatment for a first episode of unprovoked thromboembolism and after approximately 2 years of follow-up, a negative D-dimer result is associated with a 3.5% annual risk of recurrent disease, whereas a positive D-dimer result is associated with an 8.9% annual risk of recurrence. Although the role of obesity in pulmonary embolism is still unclear, the long-term risk of fatal pulmonary embolism after treatment of a venous thromboembolism may be an additional important factor in the decision to discontinue this treatment. No robust data on obese subjects are available yet.

Weight loss

Weight loss should be part of any preventive or therapeutic strategy. Weight loss is effective in reducing the risk of developing DVT. Dietary, pharmacologically, or surgically induced weight loss is effective in correcting the venous stasis disease in the majority of patients. Health-care professionals should be encouraged to emphasize the need for weight control when counseling overweight or obese patients with thrombosis. Patients of normal weight who have had a thrombosis should be advised that weight gain might increase their future risk of venous thrombosis.

Anti-coagulant therapy in obese subjects

Anti-coagulant therapy usually includes unfractionated heparin or LMWH followed by a vitamin K antagonist, administered to achieve an international normalized ratio (INR) of 2.0–3.0.

Obese patient presents potential problems for decisions regarding weight-based dosing of several anti-coagulants. Whether obese patients may need a larger thromboprophylactic dose than normo-weight patients is the subject of debate. LMWH seems to have the advantage of not requiring serial laboratory monitoring; some evidence also suggests that, compared with unfractionated heparin, LMWH decreases the risk of bleeding. Relatively few data are available concerning the dosing of LMWH in morbidly obese patients. Weight-based dosing may be preferable to fixed dosing in obese patients. However, the results are controversial and not univocal. In overweight patients, venous thromboembolism recurs more frequently with once-daily dosing of enoxaparin than with twice-daily enoxaparin dosing or intravenous unfractionated heparin. Dose capping of LMWH is not warranted, and twice-daily enoxaparin is preferred over once-daily dosing in obese patients. These differences are not statistically significant, but many clinicians believe it is prudent to choose the twice-daily regimen instead of the once-daily regimen when enoxaparin is used to treat venous thromboembolism in obese patients. In a recent study, morbidly obese patients who underwent weight-loss surgery had an incidence of DVT after surgery that was significantly lower among those given a higher-than-usual dose of LMWH than in those given a lower dose. However, another clinical study showed no significant differences in the number of thrombotic events between the usual and a higher dose of LMWH in severely obese subjects. In addition, when weight-based dosing of fondaparinux was applied, the rates of recurrent venous thrombosis embolism and major bleeding were similar regardless of weight.

Thromboembolism prophylaxis

No standardized protocols for venous thromboembolism prophylaxis in obese patients are currently available. Current prophylaxis regimens use a variety of modalities, including unfractionated heparin, LMWH, intermittent compression devices, elastic stockings, early ambulation, and an inferior vena cava filter.

Thromboembolism prophylaxis in bariatric surgery

Pulmonary embolism is a leading cause of death in bariatric patients. Thus, a venous thromboembolism prophylaxis protocol for severely obese subjects who undergo bariatric surgery has been proposed, as summarized in Figure 11.1. This venous thromboembolism prophylaxis protocol can reduce the risk of venous thromboembolism to less than 2%.

Briefly, for all patients, enoxaparin should be administered subcutaneously at 1.5 mg/kg before surgery. For all high-risk patients, post-operative warfarin therapy may be administered for 3 months. High-risk patients need increased LMWH (1.5–2.0 mg/kg twice daily) and a pre-operative inferior vena cava filter or an intraoperative intravenous heparin (1000 U/h) infusion.

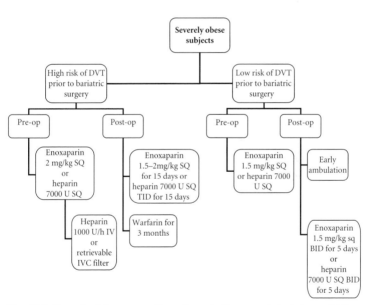

Fig. 11.1 Flow chart for venous thromboembolism prophylaxis in morbidly obese patients who undergo bariatric surgery. BID, twice daily; TID, three times daily; SQ, subcutaneously; iv, intravenously; OR, operating room. From Frezza EE & Wachtel MSI (2006) A simple venous thromboembolism prophylaxis protocol for patients undergoing bariatric surgery. *Obesity (Silver Spring)* 14:1961–65, adapted by permission from MacMillan Publishers Ltd. © 2006.

Key points

Obesity increases the risk of DVT and venous thromboembolism. Weight loss is effective in reducing the risk of developing DVT. A twice-daily regimen instead of the once-daily regimen of enoxaparin is preferred to treat venous thromboembolism in obese patients. Anti-factor Xa monitoring may be not necessary for patients weighing less than 190 kg, but can be useful for adjusting enoxaparin dosing in heavier patients.

Chapter 12

Obesity and sleep apnea

Definition of obstructive sleep apnea

Obstructive sleep apnea (OSA) is characterized by the recurrent collapse of the pharyngeal airway during sleep, which generally requires arousal to reset airway patency and resume breathing. The two major forms of OSA are:

- obstructive apnea
- obstructive hypopnea.

In obstructive apnea, upper airway obstruction is complete and therefore it may present with no airflow. In obstructive hypopnea, upper airway obstruction is partial and presents with reduction but not a complete cessation of airflow. The principle abnormality in OSA is an anatomically small pharyngeal airway. During wakefulness, the individual is able to compensate for the deficient anatomy by increasing the activity of upper airway muscles that maintain airway patency. However, with sleep onset, this compensation is lost and airway collapse occurs. The physiological consequences of apnea are a rise in the partial pressure of CO_2 in arterial blood ($PaCO_2$), a fall in PaO_2, and increased ventilatory effort against an occluded airway. Ultimately, transient arousal from sleep occurs, which resets the airway and ventilation. The individual subsequently returns to sleep and the cycle begins again, to be repeated frequently over the course of the night.

Obstructive sleep apnea and obesity

In general, obese subjects have an increased demand for ventilation and breathing workload. They can also present with respiratory muscle inefficiency, decreased functional reserve capacity and expiratory reserve volume, and closure of peripheral lung units. These dysfunctions can result in a ventilation/perfusion mismatch.

Obesity is undoubtedly the most important risk factor for OSA. Obesity is reported to be the most important demographic predictor of sleep-disordered breathing. OSA in obese subjects represents the major cause of respiratory insufficiency and pulmonary hypertension. OSA is frequently associated with morbid truncal obesity and increased visceral adiposity. The relationship between OSA and obesity is complex. Obesity causes OSA and OSA can worsen obesity. They can thus be both the cause and the consequence of each other, inducing a dangerous vicious cycle.

Obstructive sleep apnea and the obesity phenotype

The incidence of OSA increases with the severity of obesity. In fact, the prevalence among mildly or intermediately obese patients is around 30%, whereas it can be around 50–90% in morbidly obese subjects. However, recent evidence indicates that OSA is better associated with and predicted by waist circumference and waist-to-hip ratio, which are markers of central truncal adiposity, rather than by BMI. OSA can also correlate with neck size, which may increase with central obesity. Increased fat tissue deposition in the pharyngeal region can a play a role in OSA development.

Diagnosis of obstructive sleep apnea

Clinical anamnesis and ambulatory examination can often suggest OSA, particularly in morbidly obese subjects. Unfortunately, a large number of obese patients with sleep disorders can remain undiagnosed. Individuals with OSA suffer from both sleep fragmentation and the recurrent hypoxemia and hypercapnia resulting from the respiratory pause. OSA diagnosis is confirmed and diagnosed by overnight polysomnography, during which sleep is recorded while breathing, and respiratory effort, oxygen saturation, and an ECG are simultaneously monitored. Obese subjects with sleep apnea are typically characterized by an apnea–hypopnea index or respiratory disturbance index, which is the average number of apneas plus hypopneas per hour of sleep. The magnitude of oxygen desaturation is another measure commonly used to indicate the severity of the disorder.

Generally, in adults, a respiratory disturbance index of <5 is considered normal. The mild apnea range includes a respiratory disturbance index of <20 and a minimal oxygen saturation not lower than 85%, whereas the severe range includes a respiratory disturbance index of >40 or a minimal oxygen saturation of <65%.

In addition to the above respiratory tests, some cardiac examinations may be of help in assessing cardiovascular complications of OSA in obese subjects. An ECG, transthoracic echocardiogram, and cardiac catheterization may be suggested in obese subjects with suspected OSA. Echocardiography can detect functional and morphological abnormalities in the right ventricle and pulmonary arteries. ECG signs of cor pulmonale appear later than those of pulmonary hypertension assessed by right heart catheterization.

Obstructive sleep apnea and cardiovascular complications in obesity

OSA can cause several cardiovascular complications as well systemic and pulmonary hypertension, cor pulmonale, arrhythmias, myocardial infarction, right and left ventricular failure, stroke, and ultimately death. Obesity-related OSA is significantly related to systemic hypertension. The prevalence of hypertension, as well as mean systolic and diastolic blood pressure, significantly increase with increasing severity of OSA. Several mechanical, hemodynamic, and hormonal factors have been suggested to explain the association between OSA and hypertension in obese subjects. Obese subjects have a higher risk of diurnal hypertension. OSA is also correlated with insulin resistance and elevated inflammatory markers.

OSA is significantly associated with metabolic syndrome in subjects who are not necessarily obese but who present the typical increased abdominal central adiposity.

Obese subjects with OSA commonly present with pulmonary hypertension. The prevalence of pulmonary hypertension in obese subjects with OSA is around 20%. The severity of pulmonary hypertension is generally mild to moderate (pulmonary artery pressure ranging between 20 and 35 mmHg) and does not necessitate specific treatment. Pulmonary hypertension in obese subjects can increase during exercise and may be associated with hemodynamic evidence of pulmonary arteriolar hypertrophy.

Normotensive obese patients with OSA can present with increased left atrial volume index when compared with obese patients without OSA. Obese subjects with OSA usually show abnormal left ventricular diastolic function. Obese patients with OSA can also have abnormal right ventricular filling, measured by altered superior vena cava diastolic velocity during expiration.

Increased left atrial dimensions and diastolic dysfunction can lead or contribute to the development of atrial fibrillation, commonly observed in obese subjects with OSA.

Treatment of obstructive sleep apnea

The management and treatment of OSA in overweight and obese subjects should always include substantial and sustained weight loss. A 10% weight loss has been reported to potentially reduce apneic episodes by reducing the mass of the posterior airway. However, results are not univocal. Surgical weight loss is not correlated with significant resolution of OSA in morbidly obese subjects.

Continuous positive airway pressure is the first-line treatment for OSA. Other options for treating OSA include alteration of sleep posture, oral appliance therapy, external nasal support devices, and pharmacological therapy.

Surgery may sometimes be the only option. Surgical treatment options include tracheostomy, mandibular osteotomy with genioglossus or inferior border advancement, uvulopalatopharyngoplasty, laser-assisted uvuloplasty, reduction glossectomy, internal and external nasal reconstruction, tonsillectomy and adenoidectomy, and advancement of the upper and lower jaws.

Chapter 13

Weight-loss strategies

Lifestyle intervention

The primary intervention in the treatment of obese people is to achieve sustained lifestyle changes. The difficulty in achieving this goal is commonly observed in clinical practice. A combination of diet, physical activity, and behavioral therapy, including self-monitoring, goal-setting, and social support, generally result in moderate weight loss (Figure 13.1). Subsequent strategies should aim to maintain this weight loss (Figure 13.2).

Behavioral treatment

Lifestyle and behavior modifications can be facilitated by counseling from a dietician, exercise specialist, or behavioral therapist who has weight-management experience. The goal of behavioral treatment is to help obese patients identify and modify their eating habits, activity levels, and way of thinking that contribute to their excess weight. Behavioral treatment typically yields a 9–10% reduction in body weight during the first 6 months of treatment.

Dietary treatment

Reduced caloric intake is one of the cornerstones of obesity treatment. Obesity is due to (i) an imbalance in the amount of food energy consumed and the amount of energy expended through resting metabolism; (ii) the absorption, metabolism, and storage of food; and (iii) physical activity. The ideal goal is the sustained reduction of energy intake below that of energy expenditure. In fact, the rate of weight loss on a given caloric intake should be related to the rate of energy expenditure, although studies have shown that the total amount of weight lost does not correlate directly with the degree of

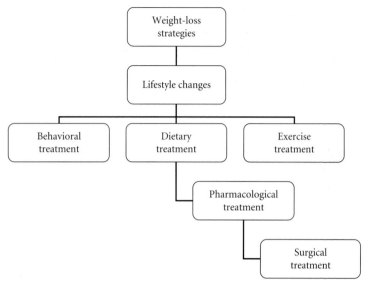

Fig. 13.1 Suggested algorithm to induce substantial weight loss.

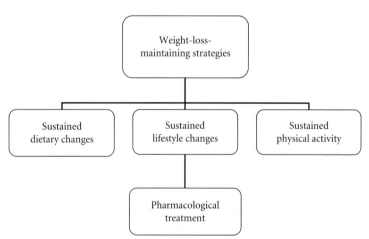

Fig. 13.2 Suggested algorithm to maintain the body weight achieved following weight loss.

energy restriction. However, chronic caloric restriction diminishes metabolic rate because of reduced lean body mass. Paradoxically, the reduction in metabolic rate with food restriction slows the rate of weight loss. A variety of different diet plans in terms of calorie content, specific food content, and form have been proposed, but there are no studies demonstrating convincingly that one type of diet is more effective and safer than another one. The degree of energy restriction of the diet appears not to have a significant impact on weight loss.

A low-energy diet recommended for the treatment of obesity should be low fat (<30%), high carbohydrate (up to 55% of daily energy intake), high protein (up to 25% of daily energy intake), and high fiber (25g/day). A high-carbohydrate, low-fat, energy-deficient diet is usually recommended for weight management by medical societies and health authorities. A moderate decrease in energy intake (−2.5 MJ/day) can result in a slow (2.5 kg/month) and sustained weight loss. To date, most studies have revealed that it is the total energy intake rather than the macronutrient composition that determines the weight loss in response to low-energy diets over a short period of time.

In spite of the generally accepted role of altered fat consumption in influencing energy balance, an agreement has not been reached concerning the effects of low-fat diets per se on weight loss. A meta-analysis of 16 dietary intervention studies demonstrated that a reduction in dietary fat without intentional restriction of energy intake caused weight loss, which was more substantial in heavier subjects. A recent lifestyle intervention study of the Diabetes Prevention Program Research Group demonstrated that, in addition to the increased physical activity, the lower percentage of calories from fat predicted weight loss over 3.2 years of follow-up. On the other hand, a meta-analysis of six randomized controlled trials specifically targeting weight loss failed to find significant differences in the effects of low-fat diets and other weight-loss diets in obese and overweight subjects. It should be noted that the ratio between saturated, monounsaturated, and polyunsaturated fatty acids in ingested fats influences metabolic and cardiovascular risks of obesity, including insulin resistance. In a recent statement, the American Diabetes Association recommended limiting the intake of saturated fats to <7% of total calories and minimizing the intake of *trans*-fat. Incorporating fish meals rich in *n*-3 fatty acids in a weight-management diet favorably affects cardiometabolic health risks including lipid profile and hypertension. However, a high intake of fish oil has been shown to moderately increase blood glucose levels and to decrease insulin sensitivity in subjects with type 2 diabetes.

Recently, the role of low-carbohydrate diets in weight management has been evaluated. These diets have been advocated because they induce many favorable effects such as rapid weight loss, a decrease in serum insulin and triglyceride levels, and a reduction in blood pressure, as well as greater suppression of appetite (partly due to ketogenesis and partly due to a higher protein intake). However, several unfavorable effects of low-carbohydrate diet administration have been demonstrated, such as increased loss of lean body mass, increased levels of low-density-lipoprotein (LDL) cholesterol and uric acid, and increased urinary calcium excretion. An extremely low intake of carbohydrate may lead to unwanted energetic efficiency. This energetic efficiency is due to the suppression of sympathetic nervous system activity and to the development of low T_3 syndrome. Long-term studies are needed to evaluate the overall changes in nutritional status, body composition, metabolic health risks, and adverse events in response to low-carbohydrate diets. Without this evaluation, low-carbohydrate diets cannot be recommended.

An increased content of protein in a diet contributes to better weight loss maintenance because proteins are more satiating and thermogenic than carbohydrates and fats. A high protein intake has been shown to sustain weight maintenance after weight loss induced by a very-low-calorie diet. Studies carried out on the role of foods with a low glycemic index and the role of increased calcium intake in reducing fat stores in human obesity have so far given conflicting results.

Dietary patterns

There are different dietary patterns. An oriental diet is considered to have a high intake of tofu and soy and other sauces. A Western diet is considered to be high in fried foods, salty snacks, eggs, and meat. A prudent diet is categorized as having a high intake of fruit and vegetables. The prudent diet is clearly associated with a reduced risk of coronary heart disease, the Western diet is weakly associated with an increased risk, and the Oriental pattern shows no significant relationship with myocardial infarction risk.

Low-calorie diets

Low-calorie diets (LCDs) >800 kcal/day are suitable for most obese patients. A diet rich in fruits, vegetables, whole grains, and other low-glycemic-index carbohydrates may promote weight loss and is preferable to low-fat diets in which large amounts of simple carbohydrates are substituted for fats. Some studies have advocated diets with protein replacement of simple carbohydrates in an effort to minimize insulin production. However, these diets have not been shown to be more effective in maintaining weight loss, and the possible long-term consequences of maintaining a lower body weight at the expense of consuming more saturated fat are unknown. Both low-fat and low-carbohydrate diets have been shown to induce weight loss and to reduce obesity-related co-morbidities. A body of evidence suggests that, although the total energy intake influences the development of obesity, the proportion of dietary energy from fat can also play a role. A recent meta-analysis suggested that reducing dietary fat is a component of successful weight maintenance. Low-carbohydrate diets cause greater short-term (up to 6 months) weight loss than low-fat diets, but the long-term clinical safety and efficacy of these diets is unknown. Increased consumption of dietary fiber can also play a role in the management of obesity through its ability to control body weight evolution through its effect on satiety. Prospective studies have also suggested that substituting whole-grain for refined-grain products may lower the risk of overweight and obesity. Meal replacements are another valid alternative dietary strategy in the treatment of obesity and have been shown to aid maintenance of weight loss in one long-term uncontrolled study.

Very-low-calorie diets

Very-low-calorie diets (VLCDs) comprising 400–600 kcal/day may be appropriate for the short-term treatment of obesity in selected patients. They are most commonly used for short periods to induce more rapid weight loss, improve co-morbidities, and provide patients with positive feedback. A very-low-energy diet consisting of 45–70 g of high-quality protein, 30–50 g of carbohydrate, and ~2 g of fat per day, as well supplements of vitamins, minerals, and trace elements, appears to be safe in selected patients under medical supervision. VLCDs contain <3.5 MJ/day and provide high-quality protein with a minor intake of fat. Vitamins, minerals, and trace elements are added to cover recommended daily allowances. VLCDs may form part of a comprehensive program undertaken by either an obesity specialist or another physician trained in nutrition and dietetics. Although the short-term weight loss induced by a VLCD is greater than that induced by standard low-calorie diets, there is no consensus on whether VLCDs per se produce greater long-term weight losses than low-calorie diets. A greater initial weight loss using VLCDs with an active follow-up weight-maintenance program, including behavioral therapy, nutrition education, and exercise, improves weight-loss maintenance. Administration of a VLCD should be limited for specific patients (i.e. those in whom rapid weight loss is indicated by a physician) and for short periods of time. Indications and contraindications for VLCD administration should be strictly followed. VLCDs should not be prescribed for patients with kidney and liver disease. However, administration of a VLCD is a reasonable approach in obese patients with type 2 diabetes. In diabetic patients treated by anti-diabetic agents, as well as in patients with hypertension treated by anti-hypertensive drugs, the drug dosage should be modified during VLCD treatment to avoid hypoglycemia or an inappropriate blood pressure decrease.

Meal-replacement diets

Meal-replacement diets (substitution of one or two daily meal portions by a VLCD) may be a useful strategy and have been shown to contribute to nutritionally well-balanced diets and weight-loss maintenance.

A meal-replacement diet may be short-term (a few weeks) or medium-term (3–6 months) programs. Obese patients are given specially formulated liquid drinks and eat specially formulated food bars. Over the next few weeks, a dietician reintroduces the patients to food. There are usually weekly support groups that patients can attend to help them maintain the weight loss.

Short-term meal-replacement programs are becoming routine in a number of bariatric surgery programs. In fact, several studies have shown that a pre-surgical meal-replacement treatment is effective in reducing body weight and improving surgical outcome in morbidly obese subjects who undergo bariatric surgery. Nutrionist and endocrinologist supervision is highly recommended.

Diets with a strict limitation of energy intake leading to semi-starvation should be strictly avoided because of serious health hazards that relate to deficiencies of several nutrients. Exaggerated lipid mobilization accompanied by an increased level of free fatty acids, together with a lack of essential amino acids and potassium and magnesium deficiencies, may promote life-threatening cardiac arrhythmias. It should be noted that obesity is frequently associated with prolongation of the QT interval, which predisposes to cardiac arrhythmias. Rapid weight loss results in an increased biliary excretion of cholesterol, which potentiates the formation of biliary stones. An increased production of ketones and ketonuria, which result from semi-starvation, prevents urinary urate excretion and leads to excessive hyperuricemia, which can result in a gout attack.

It is important to bear in mind that diets providing <5 MJ/day may yield deficiencies of several micronutrients, which could exert untoward effects not only on nutritional status but also on the weight-management outcome. It is recommended that the daily food intake is divided into four or five daily meal portions. Nutritional tables with the traffic light system can help an obese patient to choose an appropriate low-energy meal.

Key points

A low-energy diet recommended for the treatment of obesity should be low fat (<30%), high carbohydrate (up to 55% of daily energy intake), high protein (up to 25% of daily energy intake), and high fiber (25 g/day). LCDs of >800 kcal/day are suitable for most obese patients. VLCDs of 400–600 kcal/day may be appropriate for short-term treatment of obesity in selected patients. Meal-replacement treatment can be effective in reducing body weight and improving surgical outcome in morbidly obese subjects who undergo bariatric surgery.

Exercise treatment

Physical inactivity is a major modifiable risk factor for obesity. Observational evidence supports the idea that even small amounts of regular physical activity can reduce all-cause and particularly cardio-vascular mortality by 20–30%.

Exercise increases energy expenditure, stimulates fat loss, and pro-duces gains in lean muscle mass that may affect the absolute amount of weight lost. Physical activity has been reported to provide a favora-ble effect on body fat distribution. It has also been suggested that the amount of lean body mass gained through exercise is related to exer-cise intensity rather than amount. A recent Roundtable Consensus Statement from the American College of Sports Medicine reported a 'moderately strong' relationship between physical inactivity and the risk of developing obesity.

Interestingly, it has been reported that for each 1-minute improve-ment in exercise time there is a 21% reduction in the odds of gaining 10 kg. There is a dose–response relationship between the amount of weekly exercise performed and the amount of weight change in non-dieting, overweight subjects. A minimum dose of exercise equivalent to walking or jogging 10 km/week seems to be sufficient to stave off the 1 kg gained by the non-exercising controls over a 6-month period.

Exercise should be considered a crucial component of weight man-agement, although current evidence suggests exercise alone is only minimally effective in weight loss in obese subjects. In fact, several randomized controlled trials analyzed the effects of aerobic exercise without diet intervention on weight loss and concluded that it is not sufficient to have any substantial effect on weight loss without a con-current modification in diet. Randomized controlled trials have shown that aerobic exercise without diet intervention is not a very effective weight-loss strategy. However, most of these trials have some bias that may affect the results. A small randomized controlled trial showed that obese subjects who were asked to exercise enough to burn 700 kcal/day lost an average of approximately 7 kg during the 12-week study period.

In contrast, regular exercise appears to be crucial in the prevention of weight gain and successful weight-loss maintenance. Subjects with a combined diet and exercise treatment program maintained weight loss better and longer than those without exercise treatment. There is clinical evidence of better weight maintenance in subjects having a combined diet and exercise treatment compared with subjects undertaking a diet only. A large epidemiological study showed that subjects who maintained a substantial weight loss ($\geq$13.6 kg off for $\geq$1 year) used three behavioral strategies: (i) eating a diet low in fat and high in carbohydrates; (ii) frequent self-monitoring of body weight and food intake; and (iii) high levels of regular physical activity.

Most studies examining the role of exercise in the management of obesity have focused on aerobic exercise. However, a few studies have shown that resistance training has a favorable effect on body composition and metabolic profile in both overweight and obese populations.

Aerobic exercise

Aerobic physical training leads to improvements in oxygen transfer to muscles, which promotes increased utilization of abundant fat stores instead of the limited glycogen stores. Physical activity of a moderate intensity, for example 30 min in duration, performed 5 days/week is recommended. This activity conducted for a month represents an energy deficit that can contribute to 0.5 kg of weight loss. Patients should be aware of the realistic goals with regard to the expected exercise-induced weight loss as well as the beneficial effects of exercise per se on cardiometabolic risks. Obesity is usually a result of a lack of daily habitual physical activity. Therefore, activities such as walking, cycling, and stair-climbing should be encouraged. Engagement of physical activity in weight management is positively related to the level of education and inversely associated with the occurrence of serious co-morbidities, with age and with the degree of overweight. For patients with severe arthritis and problems with mobility, exercising in heated water is recommended. Vigorous physical activity that leads to joint overloading, such as jumping, should be avoided.

Strength exercise

Strength training alone is generally not considered an effective means of weight loss. Strength training usually induces significant increases in lean body mass and therefore the amount of absolute weight lost is typically unchanged or even attenuated when compared with subjects treated with diet or diet plus aerobic exercise. Strength exercises do not increase lipid oxidation but should be used, especially in less mobile disabled individuals, for protection of lean body mass and amelioration of health risks. However, because of the increased fat-free mass, resistance training has a favorable effect on body composition in obese subjects who are losing weight through dietary restriction. The diet-induced loss of fat-free mass can be almost obliterated by the addition of a combined aerobic and strength training program. The typical reduction in metabolic rate that is associated with weight loss may be counteracted by a strength training program.

Effect of exercise on obesity-related cardiovascular risk

Obese men who are cardiovascularly fit (measured by time to exhaustion on a treadmill test) have overall mortality and cardiovascular mortality rates nearly half that of normal-weight men who are unfit. Physical activity on regular basis—independent of its effect on body weight—has favorable effects on blood pressure, insulin resistance, lipid profiles and sleep apnea.

Exercise prescription in obese subjects

A minimal exercise prescription in obese subjects should include a weekly energy expenditure of at least 4200 kcal/week, the equivalent of 30 minutes or 3 km of brisk walking five times a week. More exercise may be required to induce substantial weight loss. Available data from weight-loss studies suggest that to have a significant impact on their weight, obese subjects need to burn approximately 10,500 kJ/week—the equivalent of walking or jogging 40 km/week or roughly 80 minutes of moderate aerobic activity on most days of the week.

In addition, successful weight maintenance may require expending an average of 2500 kcal/week in women and 3300 kcal/week in men, equivalent to 60–80 minutes of moderate intensity activity, such as brisk walking, on a daily basis.

Physical activity should be an integral part of comprehensive obesity management and should be individually tailored to the degree of obesity, age, and presence of co-morbidities in each subject. Physical activity not only contributes to increased energy expenditure and fat loss, but also protects against the loss of lean body mass, improves cardiorespiratory fitness, reduces obesity-related cardio-metabolic health risks, and evokes sensations of well-being.

Key points

Regular exercise appears to be crucial in the prevention of weight gain and in successful maintenance of weight loss. A minimal exercise prescription in obese subjects should include a weekly energy expenditure of at least 4200 kcal/week, the equivalent of 30 minutes or 3 km of brisk walking five times a week. Aerobic exercise is preferable in obese subjects.

Pharmacological treatment

Pharmacotherapy of obesity is indicated for the treatment of obese or overweight subjects with or without obesity-related complications.

Pharmacological therapy is indicated in individuals with a body mass index (BMI) of between 27.0 and 29.9 kg/m^2 with obesity-related medical complications, such as diabetes, metabolic syndrome, dyslipidemia, and hypertension, or in subjects with a BMI ≥30 kg/m^2.

The addition of selected pharmacological compounds to dietary and lifestyle changes is considered to induce clinically significant weight loss and an improvement in cardiometabolic risk in overweight and obese individuals with and without adiposity-related co-morbidities who are not able to achieve or maintain these goals with lifestyle changes alone.

Anti-obesity drugs have been developed to provide substantial and sustainable weight loss in combination with lifestyle changes, to improve weight loss maintenance, and to reduce obesity-related health risks. Pharmacotherapy treatment of obesity should be part of comprehensive obesity management in clinical practice.

Anti-obesity drugs affect and modulate various targets through different mechanisms and pathways. They are aimed at normalizing regulatory or metabolic adiposity-related abnormalities through central nervous system or peripheral tissue pathways. Currently, only two anti-obesity drugs, sibutramine and orlistat, have been used successfully in long-term weight management, conducted over period of 1–4 years, and are therefore approved as safe and effective medication for obesity treatment and management.

The anti-diabetic medication metformin can also be considered for weight-loss management, although its weight-loss effect is modest.

Of particular note is the anti-obesity drug rimonabant, which has been suspended recently because of the high incidence of major psychiatric issues in subjects who were taking this medication. Rimonabant is a selective endocannabinoid receptor-1 (CB-1) antagonist. Rimonabant was approved in 52 countries as an adjunct to diet and exercise for the treatment of obese patients (BMI $\geq$30 kg/m^2) or overweight patients (BMI >27 kg/m^2) with associated cardiometabolic risk factors. Although rimonabant administration was reported to induce significant weight reduction and promising improvements in cardiometabolic risk profile in four randomized double-blind clinical trials conducted in overweight or obese adults, major side effects including severe psychiatric disorders have resulted in its recent withdrawal.

Other compounds, such as adrenergic, serotonergic (suppressing appetite and food intake) and thermogenic (increasing thermogenesis) agents have recently been reported as medications for treating obesity. Nevertheless, concerns about their safety and poor evidence of their efficacy strongly discourage the use of these compounds as anti-obesity drugs.

The anti-epileptic drug topiramate has been also described to have some weight-loss effects. However, because of drug safety issues, its use as an anti-obesity agent is not recommended.

There is growing interest in the development of newer anti-obesity agents. New anti-obesity drugs with novel mechanisms of action are likely to be available in the future. Gut hormones and/or their derivatives might contribute to the treatment of obesity and provide the advantage of targeting specific appetite pathways within the brain without producing unacceptable side effects.

Key points

Pharmacological therapy is indicated in individuals with a BMI of $27.0–29.9$ kg/m^2 with obesity-related medical complications or in subjects with a BMI ≥ 30 kg/m^2. Currently approved drugs for the long-term treatment of obesity include sibutramine and orlistat.

Sibutramine

Sibutramine (sibutramine hydrochloride monohydrate) is an orally administered anti-obesity agent.

Mechanism of action

Sibutramine is a centrally acting inhibitor of serotonin and noradrenaline reuptake. Sibutramine inhibits reuptake and may stimulate the release of the biogenic amine neurotransmitters dopamine, noradrenaline and serotonin in the central nervous system and the peripheral nervous system (Figure 13.3).

Dosage

Sibutramine is available at a dose of 10 or 15 mg. The recommended starting dose is 10 mg administered once daily with or without food. If weight loss is inadequate, the dose may be titrated after 4 weeks to a dose of 15 mg once daily.

Weight-loss effect

Sibutramine is approved for the treatment of obese (BMI ≥ 30 kg/m^2) or overweight (BMI >27 kg/m^2) patients with associated cardiometabolic risk factors.

Sibutramine induces $\geq 10\%$ loss of initial body weight in almost 50% of patients or a mean difference in body weight of about 5 kg at 12 months (Figure 13.4). Sibutramine leads to weight loss by reducing hunger, enhancing satiety, and by increasing basal metabolic rate and preventing a diet-induced decline in metabolic rate.

Treatment with sibutramine results in clinically significant weight loss during short- and long-term therapy in obese adults. Sibutramine therapy can induce a more significant weight loss when given together with behavioral therapy and meal replacements.

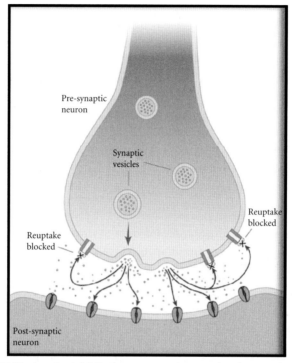

Fig. 13.3 Sibutramine inhibits the pre-synaptic reuptake of serotonin and noradrenaline.

Effects on blood pressure

Blood pressure and heart rate should be monitored closely in individuals who are taking sibutramine. Because of its central sympathomimetic action (due to enhanced noradrenaline action), in about 2% of cases sibutramine can lead to significant increases in blood pressure, particularly in diastolic blood pressure values. However, sibutramine treatment at either of the two suggested daily doses (10 or 15 mg) is unlikely to elicit a critical increase in blood pressure, even in hypertensive patients. Sibutramine should not be administered to patients with uncontrolled hypertension.

In hypertensive patients (≥140/90 mmHg) with well-controlled hypertension, a blood pressure decrease (≤5 mmHg in systolic blood

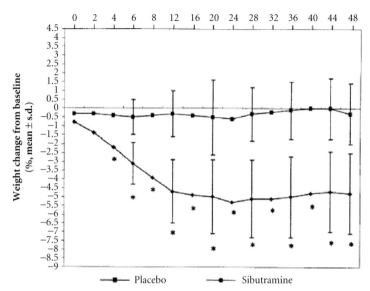

Fig. 13.4 Sibutramine induces significant weight loss compared with a placebo in obese subjects. *, Significantly different from placebo. Adapted by permission from MacMillan Publishers Ltd. Jordan J, Scholze J, Matiba B, Wirth A, Hauner H & Sharma AM (2005) Influence of sibutramine on blood pressure: evidence from placebo-controlled trials. *Int J Obes* 29, 509–16. © 2005.

pressure and ≤1 mmHg in diastolic pressure) is observed during treatment with sibutramine, even when body weight is unchanged. Concomitant anti hypertensive medication classes have not been found to affect blood pressure reductions.

In patients with normal blood pressure (≤130/85 mmHg), sibutramine-induced weight loss of >5% causes a decrease in systolic blood pressure.

A small pulse rate increase is observed with sibutramine treatment, regardless of changes in the status of blood pressure or body weight.

Effects on cardiometabolic profile

Clinical trials have shown that treatment with sibutramine can induce a significant improvement in obesity-related cardiovascular risk factors. Sibutramine can produce a significant decrease in waist circumference (about 5 cm decrease versus 1 cm decrease; $P < 0.0001$), fasting blood glucose, glycosylated hemoglobin (HbA1c), and plasma triglycerides, and an increase in HDL cholesterol when compared with the use of a placebo.

Sibutramine has been reported to induce a significant reduction in left ventricular mass in obese patients with and without hypertension.

Contraindications and side effects

Sibutramine should not be used concomitantly with serotonergic agents, including selective serotonin reuptake inhibitors, with monoamine oxidase inhibitors or with agents for migraine therapy. Caution is advised if the concomitant administration of sibutramine with other centrally acting drugs is indicated.

The most common events associated with the use of sibutramine are dry mouth, anorexia, insomnia, constipation, and headache.

Drug–drug interactions

Any drug that alters the function of dopamine, serotonin, or noradrenaline in the brain or peripheral nervous system has a strong potential for adverse interactions with sibutramine as shown in Box 13.1.

Key points

Sibutramine is a centrally acting inhibitor of serotonin and noradrenaline reuptake. A starting dose of 10 mg once daily is recommended; after 4 weeks this can be titrated to 15 mg once daily. Sibutramine induces ≥10% loss of initial body weight in almost 50% of overweight/obese patients. Blood pressure and heart rate should be monitored closely in individuals who are taking sibutramine. However, sibutramine treatment can induce a weight-loss-related decrease in blood pressure and is unlikely to cause a critical increase in blood pressure, even in hypertensive obese patients. The use of sibutramine together with lifestyle changes can improve the cardiometabolic profile and glucose control in overweight/obese subjects.

Box 13.1 Common potential drug–drug interactions with sibutramine

Selective serotonin-reuptake inhibitors
Fluoxetine, fluvoxamine, paroxetine, sertraline, venlafaxine

Monoamine oxidase inhibitors
Phenelzine, selegiline

Opioids
Dextromethorphan, meperidine, pentazocine, fentanyl, pethidine

Others
Lithium, tryptophan, ephedrine, pseudoephedrine

Anti-migraine drugs
Sumatriptan, dihydroergotamine

Cytochrome P-450 inhibitors
Ketoconazole, erythromycin, troleandomycin, cyclosporine

Cytochrome P-450 inducers
Rifampicin, phenytoin, carbamazepine, phenobarbital, dexamethasone

Orlistat

Orlistat is an orally administered anti-obesity agent.

Mechanism of action

Orlistat is a reversible lipase inhibitor for obesity management that acts by inhibiting the absorption of dietary fats. It acts in the lumen of the stomach and small intestine by forming a covalent bond with the active serine site of gastric and pancreatic lipases. The inactivated enzymes are unavailable to hydrolyze dietary fat in the form of triglycerides into absorbable free fatty acids and monoglycerides

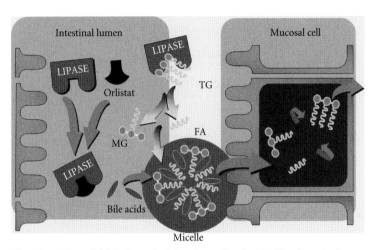

Fig. 13.5 Orlistat inhibits intestinal fat absorption by blocking intestinal lipases in obese subjects. FA, Fatty acid; MG, monoglyceride; TG, triglyceride.

(Figure 13.5). Orlistat inhibits the activity of pancreatic and gastric lipases, blocking gastrointestinal uptake of approximately 30% of ingested fat when used at a dose of 360 mg daily.

Dosage

The recommended dose of orlistat is 120 mg three times a day (360 mg daily) with each main meal. The patient should be on a nutritionally balanced LDC. Recently, the US Food and Drug Administration approved over-the-counter sale of orlistat at a dose of 60 mg three times daily.

Weight-loss effect

Orlistat is approved for the treatment of obese patients (BMI $\geq$30 kg/m^2) or overweight patients (BMI >27 kg/m^2) with associated cardiometabolic risk factors.

Orlistat may induce $\geq$10% loss of initial body weight in almost 30% of obese patients or a mean difference in body weight of about 3 kg at 12 months (Figure 13.6).

Orlistat administered for 2 years promotes weight loss and maintenance of this weight loss, and minimizes weight regain.

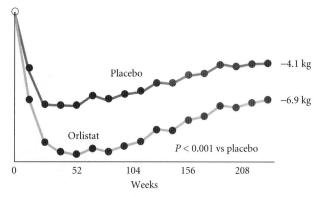

Fig. 13.6 Orlistat induces significant weight loss compared with a placebo in obese subjects.

Effects on cardiometabolic profile

Orlistat therapy improves lipid profile, glucose control, and insulin sensitivity in obese subjects with and without metabolic syndrome.

Orlistat promotes weight loss that is associated with significant reductions in blood pressure and heart rate, and may therefore have a role in the management of hypertension in overweight and obese patients.

Contraindications and side effects

Orlistat is contraindicated in patients with chronic malabsorption syndrome and cholestasis. Gastrointestinal symptoms, such as abdominal pain, diarrhea, oil spotting, and fecal urgency, are the most commonly observed side effects associated with the use of orlistat. These adverse reactions are generally mild and transient, and decrease during the second year of treatment.

Drug–drug interactions

No significant interactions between orlistat and the drugs commonly used in obese patients with cardiovascular disease have been reported. However, orlistat can interfere with the absorption of some highly lipophilic drugs, as summarized in Table 13.1.

Table 13.1 Potential drug–drug interactions with orlistat

Interaction	No interaction
Amiodarone	Atorvastatin
Warfarin	Pravastatin
	Simvastatin
	Cerivastatin
	Losartan
	Nifedipine
	Digoxin
	Metformin
	Glyburide
	Oral contraceptives

Key points

Orlistat is a reversible lipase inhibitor for obesity management that acts by inhibiting the absorption of dietary fats. The recommended dose of orlistat is 120 mg three times a day (360 mg daily) with each main meal. Orlistat may induce ≥10% loss of initial body weight in almost 30% of obese patients. Orlistat produces beneficial effects on cardiometabolic profile in overweight/obese individuals.

Metformin

Metformin hydrochloride, a dimethylbiguanidine, is currently used for the management of diabetes mellitus.

Mechanism of action

Metformin hydrochloride is an oral anti-diabetic drug that improves glucose tolerance and insulin sensitivity. Metformin decreases hepatic glucose production, decreases intestinal absorption of glucose, and improves insulin sensitivity by increasing peripheral glucose uptake and utilization.

Dosage

Metformin is an orally administered agent. Metformin hydrochloride should be given in divided doses. There is no fixed dosage regimen for treatment with metformin. The dose can be titrated from 500 mg once daily to a maximum recommended dose of 2500 mg daily.

Weight-loss effect

Metformin tends to decrease body weight in patients with obesity with and without type 2 diabetes. Long-term studies ($\geq$6 months) in drug-naive type 2 diabetic patients have demonstrated significant weight loss with metformin compared with baseline, but no significant difference when compared with a placebo.

Metformin appears to mitigate the adverse effects of insulin on body weight and induces inhibition of appetite, thus potentially explaining its mild effect on weight loss.

Metformin can be used in combination with sibutramine, orlistat, or rimonabant for weight-loss management in overweight and obese patients with dysglycemia.

Metformin can be helpful in maintaining weight loss and enhancing the metabolic and biochemical parameters achieved by treatment with sibutramine, orlistat, or rimonabant.

Effects on cardiometabolic profile

Metformin significantly improves cardiometabolic profile in overweight and obese subjects with and without diabetes.

Metformin improves metabolic parameters such as waist circumference, fasting insulin, and glucose levels, triglyceride levels in overweight and obese individuals with diabetes, glucose intolerance, impaired fasting glucose and other clinical conditions characterized by insulin resistance, and increased visceral adiposity.

Contraindications and side effects

Metformin is contraindicated in patients with renal disease or renal dysfunction, as assessed by abnormal creatinine levels and/or an abnormal glomerular filtration rate, and in patients with known acute or chronic metabolic acidosis.

Drug–drug interactions

Metformin can interact with some drugs commonly used in morbidly obese subjects as summarized in Table 13.2.

Table 13.2 Potential drug–drug interactions with metformin

Interaction	No interaction
Amiloride, furosemide, triamterene	Sulfonylureas
Calcium-channel blockers	Atenolol
Digoxin, procainamide, quinidine, quinine,	

Key points

Metformin is an oral anti-diabetic drug that improves glucose tolerance and insulin sensitivity. Metformin can be used alone or in combination with sibutramine, orlistat or rimonabant for weight-loss management in overweight and obese patients with and without diabetes. Metformin significantly improves the cardiometabolic profile in overweight and obese subjects with and without diabetes.

Glucagon-like peptide-1-based agents

Incretin hormone glucagon-like peptide-1 (GLP-1) agonists and dipeptidyl peptidase-4 (DPP4) inhibitors are a new class of anti-diabetic agent with potential weight-loss effects.

Sitagliptin (a DPP4 inhibitor) and exenatide (a GLP-1 analogue) are the only ones currently available. Others such as vildagliptin and liraglutide are currently under investigation.

Despite this, these agents are not primarily indicated for obesity and weight-loss management.

Mechanisms of action

DPP4 inhibitors and GLP-1 analogues increase insulin secretion in pancreatic β-cells in a glucose-dependent manner, suppress glucagon secretion, delay gastric emptying, and reduce appetite.

Dosage

Sitagliptin is administered orally. The recommended dose is 100 mg once daily with or without food.

Exenatide is administered by subcutaneous injection. Exenatide therapy should be initiated at 5 mcg per dose administered twice daily at any time within the 60-minute period before the morning and evening meals.

Weight-loss effect

The incretin therapies, alone or in combination with metformin and/ or thiazolidinediones, seem to improve glycemic control with the potential for weight loss in obese diabetic patients.

Orally administered DPP4 inhibitors reduce HbA1c levels by about 1%, without weight gain. The subcutaneous injected GLP-1 analogues show larger reductions in HbA1c of about 2% and weight loss (of about 3 kg) in diabetic patients. However, the long-term effects of GLP-1-based agents on weight control in obese diabetic patients has not yet been established in clinical practice.

Key points

Pharmacological treatment is approved for the treatment of obese (BMI $\geq$30 kg/m^2) or overweight (BMI >27 kg/m^2) patients with associated cardiometabolic risk factors. Sibutramine and orlistat are officially approved as anti-obesity agents and can be used in clinical practice for weight-loss management. Weight loss induced by currently available anti-obesity drugs is modest but significant, usually reaching a reduction of 5–10% of initial body weight. Interestingly, drug-induced weight loss is associated with a significant reduction in waist circumference and improvements in lipid profile and in glycemic and blood pressure control. The substantial improvement in cardiometabolic profile with anti-obesity drugs can be partly independent of weight loss. Officially approved anti-obesity medications are generally safe and well tolerated. Anti-diabetic agents, such as metformin and the new DPP4 inhibitors and GLP-1 analogues, can have some weight-loss effects in obese diabetic patients.

Bariatric surgery and cardiovascular risk

Indications for bariatric surgery

Bariatric surgery is the most effective treatment for severe and morbid obesity. Surgical treatment of obesity generally results in a more significant and longer-lasting weight loss than other treatments.

Generally, adult morbidly obese subjects may be considered for bariatric surgery when lifestyle modifications or pharmacological treatment have been inadequate to achieve a substantial and sustainable weight loss and to improve or resolve the obesity-related complications. The current indications for bariatric surgery are summarized in Box 13.2, with new criteria and recommendations expected in the near future. A possible role for bariatric surgery in subjects with complicated obesity but with a BMI lower than 35 kg/m² has been suggested and is currently under evaluation.

A summary of pre- and post-bariatric surgery management is given in Figure 13.8.

Box 13.2 Indications for bariatric surgical treatment

- BMI >40 kg/m² or >35 kg/m² with significant obesity-related co-morbidities
- Age between 16 and 65 years
- Acceptable operative risks
- Repeated failure of other non-surgical therapeutic approaches
- Psychologically stable patient with realist expectations
- Well-informed and motivated patient
- Commitment to prolonged lifestyle changes
- Supportive family/social environment
- Commitment to long-term follow-up
- Absence of alcoholism, other addictions, or major psychopathology

From the National Institutes of Health Consensus Conference (1991).

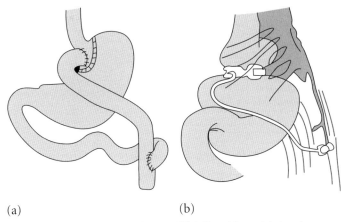

(a)   (b)

Fig. 13.7 (a) Roux-en-Y gastric bypass. (b) Adjustable gastric band.

Bariatric surgery procedures

Bariatric surgical techniques can be categorized as malabsorptive or restrictive:

- Malabsorptive procedures result in intestinal malabsorption by shortening the functional length of the intestinal surface for nutrient absorption
- Restrictive procedures result in gastric restriction, which decreases food intake by creating a small pouch and an outlet.

Biliopancreatic diversion is a malabsorptive procedure, whilst Roux-en-Y gastric bypass, biliopancreatic bypass, and duodenal switch are considered combined procedures. Each of these can be performed using a laparoscopic or open approach. Restrictive procedures include laparoscopic adjustable gastric banding and laparoscopic vertical-banded gastroplasty.

However, the most common bariatric surgical procedures performed in Europe and the USA are the laparoscopic and the laparoscopic adjustable gastric band procedures, both of which are described in Figure 13.7.

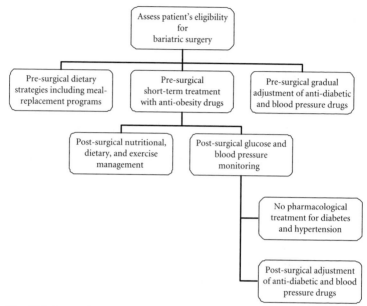

Fig. 13.8 Pre- and post-bariatric surgery management of morbidly obese subjects.

Morbidity and mortality

Mortality ranges from 0.1% for gastric banding and 0.5% for Roux-en-Y gastric bypass to 1% for biliopancreatic bypass and duodenal switch.

Laparoscopic gastric banding provides a better post-operative safety profile and therefore represents the least invasive of the frequently performed bariatric procedures. Nevertheless, these findings are not totally univocal. Laparoscopic surgery has several clinical advantages including lower surgical risk, complications, and mortality, a shorter length of stay in the hospital, and a better post-operative quality of life.

> ### Key point
> Laparoscopic adjustable gastric banding and Roux-en-Y gastric bypass are the most common bariatric surgical procedures.

Hormonal determinants of bariatric surgery-induced weight loss

Bariatric surgery induces both mechanical and hormonal changes that can explain the significant weight loss that can be achieved. The mechanisms behind these profound modifications are not completely known. Several hormones of the central nervous system, adipose tissue, and gastrointestinal tract, such as ghrelin, leptin, peptide YY, neuropeptide Y, GLP-1, pancreatic polypeptide, adiponectin, resistin, insulin, and thyroid hormones, are involved in body weight, appetite, and energy balance changes induced by bariatric surgery. The role of these hormones in predicting weight loss has been suggested, but is still not applicable in clinical practice.

Effects of bariatric surgery on body weight and cardiovascular risk

Significant weight loss (Table 13.1) and improvements in cardiovascular risk profile (Table 13.2) have been reported in morbidly obese subjects who have undergone a bariatric surgery procedure.

Weight loss

By analyzing the data from some epidemiological longitudinal studies, it was found that morbidly obese subjects who underwent bariatric surgery achieved a maximal weight loss after 1 year of about 38% (range 30–45%) with laparoscopic Roux-en-Y gastric bypass, about 22% (range 10–30%) with laparoscopic gastric banding and around 25% (range 17–25%) with laparoscopic vertical-banded gastroplasty.

Table 13.3 Effect of bariatric surgery on body fatness parameters

Changes	After 2 years*	After 10 years*
Body weight	22% decrease	16% decrease
Waist circumference	16% decrease	12% decrease
BMI	22% decrease	16% decrease

*Mean values of both laparoscopic Roux-en-Y gastric bypass and laparoscopic adjustable gastric banding.

Data adapted and simplified from Sjöström L, Lindroos AK, Peltonen M, *et al*. & the Swedish Obese Subjects Study Scientific Group (2004) Lifestyle, diabetes, and cardiovascular risk factors 10 years after bariatric surgery. *N Engl J Med* 351:2683–93.

Table 13.4 Effect of bariatric surgery on cardiovascular risk parameters

Risk parameter	After 2 years*	After 10 years*
Systolic blood pressure	3% decrease	0%
Diastolic blood pressure	3% decrease	2% decrease
Glucose	15% decrease	15% decrease
Insulin	50% decrease	30% decrease
Triglycerides	30% decrease	15% decrease
HDL cholesterol	20% increase	15% increase

*Mean values of both laparoscopic Roux-en-Y gastric bypass and laparoscopic adjustable gastric banding.

Data adapted and simplified from Sjöström L, Lindroos AK, Peltonen M, *et al.* & the Swedish Obese Subjects Study Scientific Group (2004) Lifestyle, diabetes, and cardiovascular risk factors 10 years after bariatric surgery. *N Engl J Med* 351:2683–93.

After 10 years, the maintained body weight change was around 25% (range 15–35%) in subjects who underwent gastric bypass, around 15% (range 5–25%) in individuals who underwent vertical-banded gastroplasty, and around 15% (range 5–25%) in those who had had laparoscopic gastric banding, whereas a body weight increase of around 2% (range 1–10%) occurred in obese subjects who did not undergo bariatric surgery.

Effects on regional adiposity

Bariatric surgery can induce a reduction in visceral fat mass and particularly a significant decrease in epicardial fat thickness, a marker of visceral adiposity

Effects on obesity-related co-morbidities

Bariatric surgery can improve or resolve most obesity-related co-morbidities, as well as type 2 diabetes, hypertension, and hyper-triglyceridemia. Bariatric surgery can induce complete or partial recovery from type 2 diabetes, hypertriglyceridemia, low levels of high-density lipoprotein cholesterol, hypertension, and hyperuricemia over a 2- and 10-year follow-up period.

Effects on cardiovascular risk markers

Insulin resistance and inflammatory markers significantly improve after bariatric surgery. HbA1c levels are significantly reduced after bariatric surgery, reflecting an improvement in glycemic control in obese diabetic subjects. Adiponectin levels significantly increase after bariatric surgery.

Effects on cardiac morphology and function

Bariatric surgery can induce improvements in aortic strain, distensibility, stiffness index, and both systolic and diastolic function, and a reduction in left ventricular hypertrophy. The reduction in epicardial fat thickness after bariatric surgery can be linked to morphological and functional cardiac changes.

Effects on drug therapy

The requirement for medications is generally significantly reduced after bariatric surgery.

Oral anti-diabetic agents or insulin treatment can be discontinued or significantly reduced after bariatric surgery in obese diabetic subjects. Metformin may be reintroduced because of its weight-loss effect. Insulin regimens may be adjusted to the different food intake and dietary habits that occurs after bariatric surgery. Most patients need post-operative supplements.

The blood pressure medication requirement can be different after bariatric surgery. The number of patients taking calcium-channel blockers, angiotensin-converting enzyme (ACE) inhibitors or receptor blockers, diuretics, and other agents is significantly lower after bariatric surgery.

The requirements for lipid-lowering medications can be different after bariatric surgery. Statins, ezetimibe, or fibrate use is often lower.

Post-operative adjustment of these treatments may be necessary. If conditions persist after surgery, the dosage of blood pressure medications, oral anti-diabetic agents, and insulin may be adjusted or reduced to avoid hypotension or hypoglycemic episodes.

Key points

Laparoscopic adjustable gastric banding and laparoscopic Roux-en-Y gastric bypass induce substantial and sustained weight loss and improvements in the cardiovascular risk profile in severely obese subjects. Anti-diabetic, blood pressure, and lipid-lowering therapy can be discontinued or significantly reduced after bariatric surgery. Post-operative adjustment of these treatments may be necessary.

Chapter 14

Recent trials in obesity

This chapter outlines some of the recent studies of cardiovascular risk factors in obese subjects and trials that have been carried out into the treatment of obesity using medical, surgical, and lifestyle interventions.

Risk factors

Title

'Prognostic impact of body weight and abdominal obesity in women and men with cardiovascular disease'

Aim

To assess the prognostic impact of body mass index (BMI) and abdominal obesity on cardiovascular disease patients.

Methods

Anthropometric parameters were measured in 6620 men and 2182 women, all with stable cardiovascular disease without congestive heart failure, in patients participating in the Heart Outcomes Prevention Evaluation (HOPE) study.

Outcome/results

During the 4.5-year follow-up, 658 had a cardiovascular disease-related death, 1018 had myocardial infarction, 364 had a stroke, 297 had a congestive heart failure event, and 1034 died. The adjusted relative risk of myocardial infarction in the third tertile of BMI compared with the first tertile of BMI was 20% ($P<0.02$). Similarly, the third tertile of waist circumference versus the first tertile of waist circumference had an adjusted relative risk of 23% for myocardial infarction ($P<0.01$), 38% for heart failure ($P<0.03$), and 17% for total mortality ($P<0.05$). For waist-to-hip ratio, there was an increased adjusted relative risk of 24% for cardiovascular disease-related death ($P<0.03$), 20% for myocardial infarction ($P<0.01$), and 32% for total mortality ($P<0.001$).

Conclusions

Abdominal obesity worsens the prognosis of cardiovascular disease patients.

Reference

Dagenais GR, Yi Q, Mann JF, Bosch J, Pogue J & Yusuf S (2005) *Am Heart J* 149:54–60.

Title

'Effect of potentially modifiable risk factors associated with myocardial infarction in 52 countries (the INTERHEART study): case–control study'

Aim

To identify modifiable risk factors associated with myocardial infarction in a sample representative of every inhabited continent.

Methods

Case–control study of 52 countries comprising 15152 cases and 14820 controls.

Outcome/results

Abnormal lipids, smoking, hypertension, diabetes, abdominal obesity, psychosocial factors, consumption of fruits, vegetables, and alcohol, and regular physical activity were significantly related to myocardial infarction ($P < 0.0001$ for all risk factors and $P = 0.03$ for alcohol).

Conclusions

Approaches to prevention should target the nine risk factors identified as being associated with myocardial infarction in men and women, old and young, in all regions of the world.

Reference

Yusuf S, Hawken S, Ounpuu S, *et al.* (2004) *Lancet* 364:937–52.
   'Obesity and the risk of myocardial infarction in 27,000 participants from 52 countries: a case–control study'

Title

'Obesity and the risk of myocordial infarction in 27 000 participants from 52 countries: a case control study'.

Aim

To assess whether waist-to-hip ratio (WHR) is a stronger indicator of myocardial infarction than body mass index (BMI), the conventional obesity measure.

Methods

A standardized case–control study of acute myocardial infarction was carried out with 27,098 participants in 52 countries (12,461 cases and 14,637 controls) representing several major ethnic groups.

Outcome/results

The odds ratio (OR) for the association of BMI with myocardial infarction was non-significant after adjustment of risk factors (OR 0.98, 95% CI 0.88–1.09). The OR for WHR for every successive quintile was significantly greater than that of the previous one (second quintile: 1.15, 1.05–1.26; third quintile: 1.39; 1.28–1.52; fourth quintile: 1.90, 1.74–2.07; and fifth quintile: 2.52, 2.31–2.74; adjusted for age, sex, region, and smoking).

Conclusions

WHR was found to show a graded and highly significant association with myocardial infarction risk worldwide.

Reference

Yusuf S, Hawken S, Ounpuu S, et al. (2005) Lancet 366:1640–9.

Title

'Waist circumference and waist-to-hip ratio as predictors of cardio-vascular events: meta-regression analysis of prospective studies'

Aim

To assess the association of waist circumference and waist-to-hip ratio (WHR) with the risk of incident cardiovascular disease events.

Methods

A meta-analysis was carried out of 15 prospective cohort studies or randomized clinical trials ($n = 258,114$ participants, 4355 cardiovas-cular disease events) reporting cardiovascular risk by categorical and continuous measures of waist circumference and WHR.

Outcome/results

For a 1 cm increase in waist circumference, the relative risk of a cardiovascular event increased by 2% (95% CI 1–3%) overall after adjusting for covariates. For a 0.01 unit increase in WHR, the relative risk increased by 5% (95% CI 4–7%).

Conclusions

WHR and waist circumference are associated with the risk of incident cardiovascular events.

Reference

de Koning L, Merchant AT, Pogue J & Anand SS (2007) *Eur Heart J* 28:850–6.

Medical interventions

Title

'Blood pressure changes associated with sibutramine and weight management—an analysis from the 6-week lead-in period of the Sibutramine Cardiovascular Outcomes trial (SCOUT)'

Aim

To assess changes in blood pressure and pulse associated with sibutramine use among overweight/obese patients during a 6-week lead-in period of the Sibutramine Cardiovascular Outcomes trial (SCOUT).

Methods

Analysis of changes in blood pressure and pulse after the lead-in period of a double-blind, placebo-controlled, randomized controlled trial to test sibutramine in 10,742 overweight/obese patients during which all patients received sibutramine.

Outcome/results

A blood pressure reduction [mmHg, decreased by median (5th, 95th percentile)] of –6.5 systolic (–27, 8) and –2.0 diastolic (–15, 8) was noted in the hypertensive group (50% of the 10,025 patients analyzed, who had no change in the class of anti-hypertensive medication used and who did not report an increase in anti-hypertensive medication use). When assessing the subgroup in which there was either weight gain or no weight loss, a reduction in blood pressure was also noted of –3.5 systolic (–26, 10) and –1.5 diastolic (–16, 9). All groups had an increase in pulse (1–4 b.p.m.).

Conclusions

A reduction in blood pressure was seen in all hypertensive patients over a 6-week period on sibutramine, despite no reduction in weight.

Reference

Sharma AM, Caterson ID, Coutinho W, *et al.* (2008) *Diabetes Obes Metab* 11:239–50.

Title

'Cardiovascular responses to weight management and sibutramine in high-risk subjects: an analysis from the SCOUT trial'

Aim

To assess weight changes and cardiovascular responses associated with sibutramine use among overweight/obese patients during a 6-week lead-in period of the Sibutramine Cardiovascular Outcomes (SCOUT) trial.

Methods

Analysis of changes in weight, waist circumference, and blood pressure after the lead-in period of the double-blind placebo-controlled randomized controlled trial to test sibutramine in 10,742 overweight/obese patients at increased cardiovascular risk during which all patients received sibutramine.

Outcome/results

A bodyweight reduction [median (5th, 95th percentile)] of 2.2 kg (−6.2, 0.5), waist circumference reduction of 2 cm (males: −8.5, 2.9; females: −9.0, 3.0), and reduced systolic blood pressure of 3 mmHg (−23.5, 12.5) and diastolic blood pressure of 1 mmHg (−13.5, 10.0) was observed in a high cardiovascular risk group (n = 10,742; 97% had cardiovascular disease, 88% hypertension, and 84% type 2 diabetes).

Conclusions

Sibutramine improved the cardiovascular outcomes and reduced weight in a high cardiovascular risk group of overweight and obese patients over a 6-week period.

Reference

Torp-Pedersen C, Caterson I, Coutinho W, *et al.* (2007) *Eur Heart J* 28:2915–23.

Title

'Tolerability of sibutramine during a 6-week treatment period in high-risk patients with cardiovascular disease and/or diabetes: a preliminary analysis of the Sibutramine Cardiovascular Outcomes (SCOUT) trial'

Aim

To assess the tolerability of sibutramine in a group of overweight/obese patients at increased cardiovascular risk over a 6-week lead-in period of the SCOUT trial.

Methods

Analysis of tolerability over the lead-in period of the double-blind, placebo-controlled, randomized controlled trial to test sibutramine in 10,742 overweight/obese patients at increased cardiovascular risk during which all patients received sibutramine.

Outcome/results

Of the 10,742 patients, 3.1% discontinued use due to adverse events. Serious cardiac adverse events were reported by 2.7%; however, the majority were not considered to be sibutramine-related. Increases in blood pressure and/or pulse leading to discontinuation or serious adverse events occurred in less than 0.2% of the patients. There were 15 (0.1%) deaths; ten were attributed to a cardiovascular cause.

Conclusions

Sibutramine appeared to be well tolerated in a group of overweight/obese patients at high cardiovascular risk when compared with epidemiological data.

Reference

Maggioni AP, Caterson I, Coutinho W, *et al.* (2008) *J Cardiovasc Pharmacol* 52:393–402.

Title

'Effect of orlistat on eating behavior among participants in a 3-year weight maintenance trial'

Aim

To assess dietary restraint, disinhibition, hunger, and binge eating and to understand the relationship between changes in eating behavior and weight maintenance in obese patients with metabolic syndrome.

Methods

Double-blind, orlistat/placebo-controlled, randomized controlled trial of 306 obese patients (body mass index 37.5 ± 4.1) with metabolic syndrome aged 19–45 in which an 8-week very-low-energy diet was instituted.

Outcome/results

Dietary restraint was increased and disinhibition, hunger, and binge eating decreased in both groups. The placebo group showed reduced hunger at 33 months compared with the orlistat group (difference between groups −1.1; 95% CI −2.0, −0.2; $P = 0.014$).

Conclusions

Orlistat did not affect eating behavior differently from the placebo in any substantial way in this long-term weight-maintenance trial.

Reference

Svendsen M, Rissanen A, Richelsen B, Rossner S, Hansson F & Tonstad S (2008) *Obesity (Silver Spring)* 16:327–33.

Title

'Weight loss and quality of life improvement in obese subjects treated with sibutramine: a double-blind randomized multicenter study'

Aim

To assess the efficacy of sibutramine in weight loss in obese patients.

Methods

A double-blind randomized controlled trial was carried out to compare the effect of 10 mg sibutramine with a placebo ($n = 309$) in combination with a hypocaloric diet.

Outcome/results

At 6 months, the mean weight reduction was 8.2 versus 3.9 kg in sibutramine-treated versus placebo-treated subjects, respectively ($P < 0.01$). Both sibutramine-treated (40%) and placebo-treated (14%) subjects lost ≥10% of their body weight ($P < 0.01$). Additional improvements included a reduction in body mass index (BMI) (3.1 versus 1.4 kg/m^2) and waist reduction (7.7 versus 3.5 cm) for sibutramine-treated and placebo-treated patients, respectively ($P < 0.001$). Adverse events occurred with similar low frequency in both groups.

Conclusions

Sibutramine significantly reduces weight, BMI, and waist circumference when given in conjunction with a hypocaloric diet.

Reference

Di Francesco V, Sacco T, Zamboni M, *et al.* (2007) *Ann Nutr Metab* 51:75–81.

Title
'Topical fat reduction from the waist'

Aim
To assess the effect of topical aminophylline cream on waist circumference.

Methods
Fifty participants with a body mass index (BMI) >27 kg/m² and a waist-to-hip ratio ≥1 were randomly assigned into two groups. One group applied aminophilline cream (0.05%) twice a day. All participants were instructed to participate in a walking program, to maintain a 1200 kcal/day diet and to return twice weekly.

Outcome/results
There was no change in BMI at 12 weeks. Waist circumference significantly decreased in the intervention versus the control group (11 ± 1 cm versus 5 ± 1 cm, respectively; $P<0.001$). Women lost more girth than men. No adverse events were reported. Serum aminophylline was undetectable.

Conclusions
A cosmetic reduction in local fat can be achieved by the topical use of aminophylline cream.

Reference
Caruso MK, Pekarovic S, Raum WJ & Greenway F (2007) *Diabetes Obes Metab* 9:300–3.

Title

'Long-term effects of consumption of a novel fat emulsion in relation to body-weight management'

Aim

To test the effectiveness of Olibra yoghurt versus placebo yoghurt in maintaining weight loss after a 6-week weight-loss period.

Methods

A double-blind, parallel-designed, randomized controlled trial was carried out on 50 overweight subjects ages 18–58 years (body mass index 25–32 kg/m^2). Subjects underwent an intense 6-week weight-loss program (2.1 MJ/day) prior to intervention.

Outcome/results

The placebo group increased in weight compared with the intervention group (3.0 ± 3.1 versus 1.1 ± 3.4 kg; $P < 0.001$). The test group was less hungry 4 hours after yogurt intake at week 25 ($P < 0.05$) and increased their glucagon-like peptide-1 levels 180 min after yoghurt consumption at week 25 versus week 1 of the study ($P < 0.05$). Resting energy expenditure as a function of fat-free metabolism was higher in the test group. There was a decrease in fat mass in the test group (6.5 ± 4.1 kg) compared with the placebo group (4.1 ± 3.6 kg) (week 26 versus week 2; $P < 0.05$).

Conclusions

Consumption of Olibra yoghurt improves weight maintenance.

Reference

Diepvens K, Soenen S, Steijns J, Arnold M & Westerterp-Plantenga M (2007) *Int J Obes (Lond)* 31:942–9.

Title

'Long term pharmacotherapy for obesity and overweight: updated meta-analysis'

Aim

To assess the long-term efficacy of anti-obesity drugs in weight-loss and health improvement.

Methods

An updated meta-analysis was carried out of 30 double-blind, randomized, placebo–control trials of approved anti-obesity drugs for adults. The trials for various drugs comprised: 16 for orlistat ($n = 10631$), ten for sibutramine ($n = 2623$), and four for rimonabant ($n = 6365$). These trials averaged attrition rates of 30–40%.

Outcome/results

Compared with the placebo, all of the drugs reduced weight as follows: orlistat by 2.9 kg (95% CI 2.5–3.2 kg); sibutramine by 4.2 kg (3.6–4.7 kg), and rimonabant by 4.7 kg (4.1–5.4 kg).

Orlistat resulted in a reduced incidence of diabetes, improved concentrations of total cholesterol and low-density-lipoprotein cholesterol, improved blood pressure, and glycemic control in diabetic patients. However, there were increased rates of gastrointestinal side effects and slightly lowered concentrations of high-density lipoproteins (HDLs).

Sibutramine was found to improve the concentrations of HDLs and triglycerides.

Rimonabant resulted in improved concentrations of HDLs and triglycerides, improved blood pressure, and glycaemic control in diabetic patients, but there was an increased risk of mood disorders.

Conclusions

All three medications caused moderate weight loss, and each had differing effects on cardiovascular risk profiles, as well as specific adverse effects.

Reference

Rucker D, Padwal R, Li SK, Curioni C & Lau DC (2007) BMJ 335: 1194–9.

Title

'Efficacy and safety of the weight-loss drug rimonabant: a meta-analysis of randomised trials'

Aim

To assess the safety and efficacy of the anti-obesity agent rimonabant.

Methods

A meta-analysis of four double-blind, randomized controlled trials was carried out to compare the use of 20 mg rimonabant with placebo in a total of 4105 participants.

Outcome/results

Individuals on rimonabant experienced a greater weight reduction (4.7 kg, 95% CI 4.1–5.3; $P<0.0001$) after 1 year compared with those given the placebo. However, participants on rimonabant suffered significanty more adverse events (OR = 1.4; $P = 0.0007$), serious adverse events (OR = 1.4, $P = 0.03$), depressive mood disorders (OR = 2.5; $P = 0.01$), and anxiety (OR = 3.0; $P = 0.03$) than controls.

Conclusions

Treatment with rimonabant increases the risk of severe psychiatric events. Physician alertness is required when using rimonabant.

Reference

Christensen R, Kristensen PK, Bartels EM, Bliddal H & Astrup A (2007) *Lancet* 370:1706–13.

Title

'SERENADE: the Study Evaluating Rimonabant Efficacy in Drug-naïve Diabetic Patients: effects of monotherapy with rimonabant, the first selective CB1 receptor antagonist, on glycemic control, body weight, and lipid profile in drug-naïve type 2 diabetes'

Aim

To assess the glucose-lowering efficacy and safety of rimonabant monotherapy in drug-naïve type 2 diabetic patients.

Methods

A double-blind, randomized controlled trial ($n = 281$) was carried out to compare the use of 20 mg rimonabant with placebo in drug-naïve type 2 diabetic patients.

Outcome/results

Individuals on rimonabant had a significant reduction in weight (6.7 versus 2.8 kg), waist circumference (6 versus 2 cm), plasma glucose (0.9 versus 0.1 mmol/l), and triglycerides (16.3% decrease versus 4.4% increase from baseline). The intervention group also experienced increased high-density-lipoprotein cholesterol (10.1 versus 3.2%), dizziness (10.9 versus 2.1%), nausea (8.7 versus 3.6%), anxiety (5.8 versus 3.6%), depressed moods (5.8 versus 0.7%), and paresthesia (2.9 versus 1.4%) compared with controls.

Conclusions

Rimonabant improves glycemic control, body weight, and lipid profile in drug-naïve type 2 diabetic patients. However, further studies are needed to determine the risk-to-benefit profile.

Reference

Rosenstock J, Hollander P, Chevalier S, Iranmanesh A & the SERENADE Study Group (2008) *Diabetes Care* 31:2169–76.

Title

'Effect of rimonabant on progression of atherosclerosis in patients with abdominal obesity and coronary artery disease: the STRADI-VARIUS randomized controlled trial'

Aim

To assess whether the weight loss and metabolic effects of rimonabant decrease the progression of coronary disease.

Methods

A randomized, double-blind, placebo-controlled, two-group, parallel-group trial ($n = 839$) was carried out to compare the use of 20 mg rimonabant with placebo in patients with abdominal obesity and metabolic syndrome.

Outcome/results

Compared with the placebo group, the rimonabant group had a reduced percentage atheroma volume (PAV) (0.25% versus 0.51%; $P = 0.22$)) and total atheroma volume (TAV) (2.2 versus 0.88 mm^3; $P = 0.03$). The intervention group also demonstrated weight reduction (4.3 kg versus 0.5 kg with placebo), a reduced waist circumference (4.5 cm reduction versus 1.0 cm with placebo), decreased triglycerides (20.5 versus 6.2%), increased high-density-lipoprotein cholesterol (22.4 versus 6.9%) and an increase in psychiatric effects (43.4 versus 28.4%).

Conclusions

Although the study failed to reveal an effect of rimonabant on the progression of coronary disease for the primary end-point (PAV), a favorable effect for the secondary end-point (TAV) was revealed. Further studies are needed to assess whether rimonabant is useful in managing coronary disease.

Reference

Nissen SE, Nicholls SJ, Wolski K, *et al.* (2008) *JAMA* 299:1547–60.

Title

'Long-term effect of CB1 blockade with rimonabant on cardiometabolic risk factors: two year results from the RIO-Europe Study'

Aim

To assess the efficacy of rimonabant on weight loss and improvement of cardiometabolic risk factors over a 2-year period.

Methods

A double-blind, randomized controlled trial was carried out to compare the use of 5 or 20 mg of rimonabant once daily with placebo in patients with a body mass index ≥ 30 or > 27 kg/m^2 with untreated hypertension, dyslipidemia, or both, on a calorie-restricted diet for 2 years.

Outcome/results

A weight reduction was seen (mean ± SD: –5.5 ± 7.7 kg; $P < 0.001$) in participants given 20 mg (–2.9 ± 6.5 kg; $P = 0.002$) or 5 mg (–1.2 ± 6.8 kg) rimonabant versus placebo. Additional improvements with 20 mg rimonabant included waist circumference reduction, improved levels of high-density lipoproteins, triglycerides, fasting glucose and insulin, insulin resistance, and metabolic syndrome prevalence. During the second year, the rates of adverse events including depressive mood disorders and disturbances were similar to those seen in the placebo group.

Conclusions

Over a 2-year period, administration of 20 mg rimonabant resulted in clinically significant weight loss and improvements in cardiometabolic risk factors.

Reference

Van Gaal LF, Scheen AJ, Rissanen AM, Rossner S, Hanotin C & Ziegler O (2008) *Eur Heart J* 29:1761–71.

Surgical interventions

Title

'Maximal weight loss after banded and unbanded laparoscopic Roux-en-Y gastric bypass: a randomized controlled trial'

Aim

To compare the effectiveness and safety of banded verses unbanded laparoscopic Roux-en-Y gastric bypass.

Methods

A pilot randomized controlled trial was carried out using 60 patients divided into two groups of 30. No significant differences existed between the two groups in terms of age, gender, body mass index (BMI), or operative time.

Outcome/results

BMI and weight loss were similar among the two groups at 6, 12, and 24 months. The complication rates were also similar.

Conclusions

There were insignificant differences in maximal weight loss, mortality, and morbidity between the two procedures. Further long-term studies are necessary to assess weight maintenance and regain using these methods.

Reference

Arceo-Olaiz R, España-Gómez MN, Montalvo-Hernández J, Velázquez-Fernández D, Pantoja JP & Herrera MF (2008) *Surg Obes Relat Dis* 4:507–11.

Title

'Weight loss, appetite suppression, and changes in fasting and post-prandial ghrelin and peptide-YY levels after Roux-en-Y gastric bypass and sleeve gastrectomy: a prospective, double blind study'

Aim

To compare the effectiveness of laparoscopic sleeve gastrectomy (LSG) and laparoscopic Roux-en-Y gastric bypass (LRYGB).

Methods

A prospective double-blind, randomized controlled trial ($n = 32$) was carried out to compare the use of LSG ($n = 16$) with LRYGB ($n = 16$). Follow-up was at 1, 3, 6, and 12 months.

Outcome/results

There was a significant reduction in body weight and an increase in peptide-YY in both groups. There was greater weight loss in the LSG group at 6 months (55.5 ± 7.6 versus $50.2 \pm 6.5\%$; $P = 0.04$) and 12 months (69.7 ± 14.6 versus $60.5 \pm 10.7\%$; $P = 0.05$). Ghrelin levels and appetite were significantly suppressed in the LSG group.

Conclusions

LSG results in greater appetite and ghrelin suppression, as well as weight loss.

Reference

Karamanakos SN, Vagenas K, Kalfarentzos F & Alexandrides TK (2008) *Ann Surg* 247:401–7.

Title

'Safety and effectiveness of the intragastric balloon for obesity—a meta-analysis'

Aim

To assess the safety, efficacy, and effectiveness of the BioEnterics Intragastric Balloon (BIB) for the treatment of obesity.

Methods

A meta-analysis of weighted mean difference was carried out using the inverse variance method ($n = 3608$).

Outcome/results

At balloon removal, the estimates for weight loss were as follows: 14.7 kg, 12.2% of initial weight, 5.7 kg/m^2, and 32.1% of excess weight. After balloon removal, a meta-analysis of two randomized controlled trials ($n = 75$) show a greater weight loss among balloon-treated patients (6.7 kg, 1.5% of initial weight, 3.2 kg/m^2, and 17.6% of excess weight) than placebo-treated patients. Early removal of the BIB occurred in 4.2% of cases and most complications were mild.

Conclusions

The study revealed that BIB, when used with a weight-management program, is effective for weight loss in the short term. Long-term maintenance of weight loss using this technique is unknown.

Reference

Imaz I, Martínez-Cervell C, García-Alvarez EE, Sendra-Gutiérrez JM & González-Enríquez J (2008) *Obes Surg* 18:841–6.

Title

'A prospective randomized study comparing two different techniques for laparoscopic sleeve gastrectomy'

Aim

To compare two techniques of performing laparoscopic sleeve gastrectomy (LSG).

Methods

A prospective randomized controlled trial was carried out to compare two techniques of performing LSG. Group A ($n = 20$) used a technique where stapling was performed after full devascularization and mobilization of the gastric curve. Group B ($n = 20$) used a technique where stapling was performed as soon as the lesser sac was entered, and the greater curve was devascularized after full completion of the sleeve.

Outcome/results

The median operative times were 34 min (12–54) for group A and 25 min (9–51) for group B ($P = 0.06$). The median pre-operative bleeding was 5 ml (0–450) for group A and 5 m (0–100) for group B ($P = 0.37$). The median number of staple cartridges was six (five to seven) for group A and six (four to seven) for group B ($P = 0.63$). The following features were also noted:

- Peroperative complications: small hiatal hernia requiring repair and bleeding in two group A patients
- Postoperative leak: in one group A patient
- Minor early complications: two in group A patients and one in a group B patient
- Median hospital stay: 3 days (1–10) for group A and 3 days (2–7) for group B ($P = 0.59$)
- Late complication: stenosis in one group B patient
- Excess weight loss: 43.4% for group A and 42.2% for group B at 6 months; 48.3% for group A and 49.5% for group B at 12 months ($P = 0.82$).

Conclusions

No significant differences were found between the two techniques. For the observed distributions, group B had better results than group A with respect to hospital stay, operative time, and pre-operative bleeding.

Reference

Dapri G, Vaz C, Cadière GB & Himpens J (2007) *Obes Surg* 17:1435–41.

Lifestyle interventions

Title

'Alteration of dietary fat intake to prevent weight gain: Jayhawk Observed Eating Trial'

Aim

To compare the effect of the amount of dietary fat intake on weight gain.

Methods

A randomized trial was carried out of 305 participants, divided into three groups: low fat intake (<25% of total energy), medium fat intake (28–32% of total energy), and high fat intake (>35% of total energy). The study period was 12 weeks.

Outcome/results

Most of the participants completed the study ($n = 260$). The low-fat group gained 0.1 ± 3.1 kg, the medium-fat group gained 0.8 ± 2.5 kg, and the high-fat group gained 1.0 ± 2.2 kg. However, adjusting for total energy intake eliminated any differences in effect on weight gain.

Conclusions

Total energy intake, rather than the percentage of energy from fat, is responsible for weight gain. However, a low-fat versus a high-fat diet may influence total energy intake.

Reference

Donnelly JE, Sullivan DK, Smith BK, *et al.* (2008) *Obesity (Silver Spring)* 16:107–12.

Title

'Body fat loss achieved by stimulation of thermogenesis by a combination of bioactive food ingredients: a placebo-controlled, double-blind 8-week intervention in obese subjects'

Aim

To test the effect of a combination of tyrosine, capsaicin, catechines, caffeine and calcium on weight loss, thermogenesis, fecal fat excretion, blood pressure, and heart rate.

Methods

A double-blind, randomized controlled trial was carried out to test an 8-week bioactive ingredient intervention compared with a placebo in 80 overweight/obese [body mass index 31.2 ± 2.5 kg/m^2 (mean $\pm$ SD)] individuals who had lost >4% of their body weight (6.9 ± 1.9 kg) in an earlier 4-week hypocaloric trial.

Outcome/results

There was a weight reduction of 0.9 kg in the intervention group. Thermogenesis was 87.3 kJ/4 h (95% CI 50.9–123.7; $P = 0.005$) compared with the placebo at the start of the trial. After 8 weeks, this effect was sustained (85.5 kJ/4 h, 95% CI 47.6–123.4; $P = 0.03$). No change in heart rate, blood pressure, or fecal fat excretion was found.

Conclusions

Bioactive intervention may allow sustained weight loss in individuals who undertake a hypocaloric diet.

Reference

Belza A, Frandsen E & Kondrup J (2007) *Int J Obes (Lond)* 31: 121–30.

Title

'The role of conjugated linoleic acid in reducing body fat and preventing holiday weight gain'

Aim

To test the effect of conjugated linoleic acid on body fat and the prevention of weight gain.

Methods

A double-blind randomized controlled trial was carried out in 40 healthy, overweight individuals (body mass index 25–30 kg/m^2) comparing the use of conjugated linoleic acid (3.2 g/day) with placebo over a 6-month intervention period.

Outcome/results

The placebo group gained weight compared with the intervention group during the November–December (holiday) period ($P = 0.01$). Body fat was significantly reduced in the conjugated linoleic acid group over the 6-month period (-1.0 ± 2.2 kg; $P = 0.05$).

Conclusions

Conjugated linoleic acid supplementation among overweight adults significantly reduced body fat over a period of 6 months and prevented weight gain during the holiday season. Studies investigating the safety of prolonged use of conjugated linoleic acid are necessary.

Reference

Watras AC, Buchholz AC, Close RN, Zhang Z & Schoeller DA (2007) *Int J Obes (Lond)* 31:481–7.

Title

'Efficacy of conjugated linoleic acid for reducing fat mass: a meta-analysis in humans'

Aim

To assess the efficacy of conjugated linoleic acid in reducing fat mass.

Methods

A meta-analysis was carried out of double-blind, placebo-controlled, randomized studies assessing the use of conjugated linoleic acid and body composition reduction (measured by a validated technique). Of 18 identified studies, 15 were included (three did not present sufficient information for the conjugated form).

Outcome/results

A linear weight loss was seen over 6 months that approached an asymptote at 2 years. With a dose of 3.2 g/day, there was a reduction in fat mass for the conjugated linoleic acid group alone (0.05 ± 0.05 kg/week; $P < 0.001$) and for the conjugated linoleic acid group compared with the placebo (0.09 ± 0.08 kg/week; $P < 0.001$).

Conclusions

Conjugated linoleic acid promotes moderate body fat reduction.

Reference

Whigham LD, Watras AC & Schoeller DA (2007) *Am J Clin Nutr* 85:1203–11.

Title

'Weight loss with a low-carbohydrate, Mediterranean, or low-fat diet'

Aim

To compare and assess the efficacy of three diets: low carbohydrate, Mediterranean, and low fat.

Methods

A randomized controlled comparative study was carried out to compare weight loss based on three diets (low carbohydrate, unrestricted calories; Mediterranean, restricted calories; and low fat, restricted calories) on randomly assigned, moderately obese subjects ($n = 322$).

Outcome/results

The mean weight loss observed was 2.9 kg for the low-fat diet, 4.4 kg for the Mediterranean diet, and 4.7 kg for the low-carbohydrate diet ($P<0.001$ for the interaction between diet group and time). For those who completed the intervention, the mean weight loss was 3.3 kg for the low-fat diet, 4.6 kg for the Mediterranean diet, and 5.5 kg for the low-carbohydrate diet.

The reduction in the ratio of total cholesterol to high-density-lipoprotein cholesterol was 12% in the low-fat-diet group and 20% in the low-carbohydrate-diet group ($P = 0.01$).

Changes in fasting plasma glucose and insulin levels among diabetic patients were more favorable in the Mediterranean diet group than the low-fat diet group ($P<0.001$ for the interaction among diabetes and Mediterranean diet and time with respect to fasting glucose levels.

Conclusions

Both low-carbohydrate and Mediterranean diets may be effective substitutes for low-fat diets. The Mediterranean diet provided a more favorable effect on glycemic control, whilst the low-carbohydrate diet provided a more favorable effect on lipids.

Reference

Shai I, Schwarzfuchs D, Henkin Y, *et al.* (2008) *N Engl J Med* 359:229–41.

Title

'Family dietary coaching to improve nutritional intakes and body weight control: a randomized control trial'

Aim

To assess whether family dietary coaching improves nutritional intake and weight control in non-institutionalized parents and children.

Methods

A randomized controlled trial was carried out comparing three groups of parents (total $n = 1013$) and children (total $n = 1013$): group A was advised to reduce their fat and increase their complex carbohydrate intake; group B was advised to reduce both fat and sugar and to increase complex carbohydrate intake; and the control group was given no advice. Groups A and B were counseled monthly by phone and monitored on the Internet for 8 months.

Outcome/results

Groups A and B both decreased their energy intake, reaching their nutritional targets for fat intake and to a lesser extent for sugar and complex carbohydrates (children, $P < 0.001$; parents, $P = 0.02$).

The mean changes in body mass index (BMI, kg/m^2) differed among parents (group A: +0.13, 95% CI –0.01 to 0.27; group B: –0.02, 95% CI, –0.14 to 0.11; control group: +0.24, 95% CI 0.13 to 0.34; $P = 0.001$) with a significant difference between group B and the control group ($P = 0.01$).

In contrast, the mean changes in BMI were similar for the children (group A: +0.05, 95% CI –0.06 to 0.16; group B: +0.10, 95% CI –0.03 to 0.23; control group: +0.13, 95% CI 0.04 to 0.22; $P = 0.45$).

Conclusions

Family dietary coaching improves the nutritional intake for non-institutionalized parents and children, and also improves weight control for parents.

Reference

Paineau DL, Beaufils F, Boulier A, *et al.* (2008) *Arch Pediatr Adolesc Med* 162:34–43.

Exercise

Title

'Effect of exercise on 24-month weight loss maintenance in overweight women'

Aim

To assess the efficacy of non-surgical interventions in pediatric obesity.

Methods

A randomized controlled comparative study was carried out to compare the effect of moderate versus rigorous exercise in combination with high- versus moderate-duration exercise on overweight and obese women ($n = 201$).

Outcome/results

Weight loss in the randomized groups at 6 months (8–10% of initial body weight) and 24 months (5% of initial body weight) was similar. However, maintenance of loss of ≥10% of initial body weight at 24 months occurred in individuals performing more physical activity (1835 kcal/week or 275 min/week) than those maintaining a weight loss of <10% of initial body weight ($P < 0.001$).

Conclusions

This study suggests that, to maintain a weight loss of >10%, overweight women should carry out 275 min/week of physical activity along with reducing energy intake.

Reference

Jakicic JM, Marcus BH, Lang W & Janney C (2008) *Arch Intern Med* 168:1550–9; discussion 1559–60.

Title

'A meta-analysis of pedometer-based walking interventions and weight loss'

Aim

To assess whether pedometer-based walking programs encouraging increased step counts result in weight loss.

Methods

A meta-analysis and review was carried out of nine randomized controlled trials with a cohort sample size ranging from 15 to 106 for a total of 307 overweight or obese sedentary participants. Intervention duration ranged from 4 weeks to 1 year (median duration of 16 weeks).

Outcome/results

During the interventions, individuals lost 0.05 kg/week, and the weight change was greater with a longer intervention duration.

Conclusions

Pedometer-based programs result in moderate weight loss, with longer programs resulting in greater weight loss.

Reference

Richardson CR, Newton TL, Abraham JJ, Sen A, Jimbo M & Swartz AM (2008) *Ann Fam Med* 6:69–77.

Combined/other methods

Title

'Weight-loss outcomes: a systematic review and meta-analysis of weight-loss clinical trials with a minimum 1-year follow-up'

Aim

To assess the efficacy of weight-loss interventions and to identify expected weight-loss outcomes resulting from such interventions.

Methods

A meta-analysis and review was carried out of 80 randomized clinical trials with ≥1 year follow-up. Eight types of weight-loss intervention were identified: diet alone, diet and exercise, exercise alone, meal replacements, very-low-energy diets, weight-loss medications (orlistat or sibutramine), and advice alone.

Outcome/results

For the reduced-energy diet and/or weight-loss medications, there was a mean weight loss of 5–8.5 kg (5–9%) with weight plateauing at approximately 6 months. At 48 months, a mean 3–6 kg (3–6%) weight loss was maintained with no weight regain to baseline.

For the advice-only and exercise-alone groups, there was minimal weight loss at any given time.

Conclusions

A reduced-energy diet and exercise interventions resulted in moderate weight loss at 6 months with general maintenance of weight despite some regain. Weight-loss medications improve the maintenance of weight loss.

Reference

Franz MJ, VanWormer JJ, Crain AL, *et al.* (2007) *J Am Diet Assoc* 107:1755–67.

Title

'Maintenance of weight loss in overweight middle-aged women through the Internet'

Aim

To compare the weight regain among two groups of peri-menopausal women after a 4-month weight-loss treatment: those with 12-month weight maintenance Internet intervention and those with self-directed weight maintenance.

Methods

A randomized controlled comparative study was carried out between two groups of peri-menopausal women ($n = 135$) following a 4-month behavioral weight-loss program: an Internet intervention group ($n = 66$) and a self-directed group ($n = 69$). Both groups were interviewed using 7-day physical activity questionnaires at baseline, 4 months, and 16 months.

Outcome/results

At 12 months, the Internet group had regained an average of 0.4 ± 5.0 kg, whilst the self-directed group had regained an average of 0.6 ± 4.0 kg ($P = 0.5$).

Internet diet log entries correlated with weight change ($r = -0.29$, $P < 0.05$) and change in exercise energy expenditure ($r = 0.44$, $P < 0.01$).

Conclusions

Both groups maintained significant weight loss, and the Internet group did not surpass the self-directed group in weight-loss maintenance.

Reference

Cussler EC, Teixeira PJ, Going SB, et al. (2008) Obesity (Silver Spring) 16:1052–60.

Title

'Comparison of strategies for sustaining weight loss: the weight loss maintenance randomized control trial'

Aim

To compare two weight-loss-maintenance interventions (personal contact and interactive technology) with a self-directed control group.

Methods

A comparative, multi-center, randomized controlled trial was carried out. Following a weight-loss program, participants were randomly assigned to three groups with monthly personal contact, unlimited access to an interactive technology-based program or under self-directed control.

Outcome/results

Weight regain occurred in all groups, but the personal-contact group regained less weight (4.0 kg) than the self-directed group (5.5 kg; mean difference at 30 months, -1.5 kg; 95% CI -2.4 to -0.6 kg; $P = 0.001$).

At 30 months there was no difference in weight regain between the interactive technology-based (5.3 kg) and self-directed groups (5.5 kg; mean difference -0.3 kg; 95% CI -1.2 to 0.6 kg; $P = 0.51$); however, at 18 and 24 months weight, regain was lower in the interactive technology-based group than in the self-directed group: mean difference at 18 months, -1.1 kg; 95% CI -1.9 to -0.4 kg; $P = 0.003$); 24 months (mean difference, -0.9 kg; 95% CI -1.7 to -0.02 kg; $P = 0.03$).

The difference between the personal-contact and interactive technology-based group at 30 months was -1.2 kg (95% CI -2.1 to -0.3; $P = 0.008$).

Of all the study participants, 71% maintained a weight below their initial level.

Conclusions

Most study participants maintained a lower-than-entry-level weight. The interactive technology-based group provided an early but transient benefit, whilst monthly brief personal contact provided a modest benefit in weight-loss maintenance.

Reference

Svetkey LP, Stevens VJ, Brantley PJ, *et al.* (2008) *JAMA* 299:1139–48.

Title

'Randomized, controlled trial of an internet facilitated intervention for reducing binge eating and overweight in adolescents'

Aim

To determine the efficacy of an Internet-facilitated intervention for binge eating and weight maintenance in adolescents.

Methods

A randomized controlled trial was carried out to compare weight maintenance and binge eating between two groups of adolescent students: StudentBodies2-BED ($n = 52$), a 16-week online intervention, and a wait-list control group ($n = 53$), at three time points: baseline, post-treatment, and follow-up.

Outcome/results

From baseline to follow-up, the StudentBodies2-BED group had significantly lower body mass index (BMI) z scores and BMI than the wait-list control group. The StudentBodies2-BED group also had significantly lower objective as well as subjective binge episodes from both baseline to post-treatment and baseline to follow-up.

In the StudentBodies2-BED group, there were fewer weight/shape concerns from post-treatment to follow-up and from baseline to follow up, and a lower BMI at follow-up among those who engaged in objective binge-eating episodes at baseline.

Conclusions

Although only moderately effective in short-term weight loss and maintenance, an Internet-facilitated intervention is very effective in significantly reducing binge eating.

Reference

Jones M, Luce KH, Osborne MI, *et al.* (2008) *Pediatrics* 121:453–62.

Title

'Effect of lifestyle intervention on the occurrence of metabolic syndrome and its components in the Finnish Diabetes Prevention Study'

Aim

To assess the effect of lifestyle intervention on metabolic syndrome (as defined by the National Cholesterol Education Program 2005).

Methods

A secondary analysis was carried out of the Finnish Diabetes Prevention Study of overweight (body mass index 31.2 ± 4.6 kg/m^2), middle-aged (55 ± 7 years) men ($n = 172$) and women ($n = 350$) with impaired glucose tolerance. A randomized trial was conducted to compare the intervention ($n = 265$) and control ($n = 257$) groups.

Outcome/results

There was a mean follow-up of 3.9 years. The prevalence of metabolic syndrome had decreased from 74 to 62.6% in the intervention group and from 74 to 71.2% in the control group by the end of the study (odds ratio 0.62, 95% CI 0.40–0.95). Abdominal obesity was also relatively decreased (prevalence of abdominal obesity: odds ratio 0.48, 95% CI 0.28–0.81).

Conclusions

Lifestyle intervention reduces the risk of metabolic syndrome in middle-aged, overweight, glucose-impaired patients.

Reference

Ilanne-Parikka P, Eriksson JG, Lindstrom J, *et al.* (2008) *Diabetes Care* 31:805–7.

Title

'Treatment of pediatric obesity. A systematic review and meta-analysis of randomized trials'

Aim

To assess the efficacy of non-surgical interventions on pediatric obesity.

Methods

A meta-analysis and review was carried out of 61 randomized controlled trials of overweight children and adolescents.

Outcome/results

There was a reduction in body mass index (BMI) with the use of sibutramine (2.4 kg/m^2) and orlistat (0.7 kg/m^2).

Physical activity was found to have a moderate effect on adiposity (effect size -0.52, 95% CI -0.73 to -0.30), whilst no significant effect was revealed on BMI (effect size -0.02, 95% CI -0.21 to 0.18). However, this finding may be the result of reporting bias.

Twenty-four trials measuring combined lifestyle interventions revealed only small changes in BMI.

Conclusions

Medications and lifestyle interventions result in short-term efficacy in treating pediatric obesity; however, the supporting evidence is limited.

Reference

McGovern L, Johnson JN, Paulo R, *et al.* (2008) *J Clin Endocrinol Metab* 93:4600–5.

Bibliography

Obesity cardiovascular risk

Anand SS, Yusuf S, Vuksan V, *et al.* (2000) Differences in risk factors, atherosclerosis, and cardiovascular disease between ethnic groups in Canada: the Study of Health Assessment and Risk in Ethnic groups (SHARE). *Lancet* 356:279–84.

Baik I, Ascherio A, Rimm EB, *et al.* (2000) Adiposity and mortality in men. *Am J Epidemiol* 152: 264–71.

Despres JP & Lemieux I (2006) Abdominal obesity and metabolic syndrome. *Nature* 444:881–7.

Expert Panel on Detection, Evaluation, and Treatment of High Blood Cholesterol in Adults (2001). Executive summary of The Third Report of The National Cholesterol Education Program (NCEP) Expert panel on Detection, Evaluation, and Treatment of High Blood Cholesterol in Adults (Adult Treatment Panel III). *JAMA* 285:2486–97.

Fox CS, Massaro JM, Hoffmann U, *et al.* (2007) Abdominal visceral and subcutaneous adipose tissue compartments: association with metabolic risk factors in the Framingham Heart Study. *Circulation* 116:39–48.

Kragelund C, Hassager C, Hildebrandt P, Torp-Pedersen C, Kober L & the TRACE study group. (2005) Impact of obesity on long-term prognosis following acute myocardial infarction. *Int J Cardiol* 98:123–31.

Kuk JL, Katzmarzyk PT, Nichaman MZ, Church TS, Blair SN & Ross R (2006) Visceral fat is an independent predictor of all-cause mortality in men. *Obes Res* 14:336–41.

Misra A & Vikram NK (2003) Clinical and pathophysiological consequences of abdominal adiposity and abdominal adipose tissue depots. *Nutrition* 19:457–66.

National Institutes of Health (1998) Clinical guidelines on the identification, evaluation, and treatment of overweight and obesity in adults: the evidence report. *Obes Res* 6 (Suppl. 2): 51S–209S.

Poirier P, Giles TD, Bray GA, *et al.* (2006) Obesity and cardiovascular disease: pathophysiology, evaluation, and effect of weight loss: an update of the 1997 American Heart Association Scientific Statement on Obesity and Heart Disease from the Obesity Committee of the Council on Nutrition, Physical Activity, and Metabolism. *Circulation* 113:898–918.

Romero-Corral A, Montori VM, Somers VK, *et al.* (2006) Association of bodyweight with total mortality and with cardiovascular events in coronary artery disease: a systematic review of cohort studies. *Lancet* 368:666–78.

Smith SR (2006) Importance of diagnosing and treating the metabolic syndrome in reducing cardiovascular risk. *Obesity (Silver Spring)* 14 (Suppl. 3): 128S–134S.

Sowers, JR (2003) Obesity as a cardiovascular risk factor. *Am J Med* 8 (Suppl. 8A), 37S–41S.

Wilson PW, D'Agostino RB, Sullivan L, Parise H & Kannel WB (2002) Overweight and obesity as determinants of cardiovascular risk: the Framingham experience. *Arch Intern Med* 162,1867–72.

Yusuf S, Hawken S, Ounpuu S, *et al.* (2005) Obesity and the risk of myocardial infarction in 27,000 participants from 52 countries: a case–control study. *Lancet* 366:1640–9.

Metabolic syndrome

Aguilar-Salinas CA, Rojas R, Gómez-Pérez FJ, *et al.* (2003) Analysis of the agreement between the World Health Organization criteria and the National Cholesterol Education Program-III definition of the metabolic syndrome: results from a population-based survey. *Diabetes Care* 26: 1635.

Alberti KG & Zimmet PZ (1998) Definition, diagnosis and classification of diabetes mellitus and its complications: Part 1. Diagnosis and classification of diabetes mellitus provisional report of a WHO consultation. *Diabet Med* 15: 539–53.

Balkau B, Charles MA, Drivsholm T, *et al.* (2002) Frequency of the WHO metabolic syndrome in European cohorts, and an alternative definition of an insulin resistance syndrome. *Diabetes Metab* 28: 364–76.

Bonora E, Targher G, Formentini G, *et al.* (2004) The Metabolic Syndrome is an independent predictor of cardiovascular disease in Type 2 diabetic subjects. Prospective data from the Verona Diabetes Complications Study. *Diabet Med* 21:52–58.

Expert Panel on Detection, Evaluation, and Treatment of High Blood Cholesterol in Adults (2001) Executive Summary of The Third Report of The National Cholesterol Education Program (NCEP) Expert Panel on Detection, Evaluation, and Treatment of High Blood Cholesterol in Adults (Adult Treatment Panel III). *JAMA* 285:2486–97.

Ford ES, Giles WH & Dietz WH (2002) Prevalence of the metabolic syndrome among US adults: findings from the third national health and nutrition examination survey. *JAMA* 287:356–9.

Ford ES, Giles W & Mokdad A (2004) Increasing prevalence of the metabolic syndrome among US adults. *Diabetes Care* 27:2444–9.

Groop L & Orho-Melander M (2001) The dysmetabolic syndrome. *J Intern Med* 250:105–20.

Grundy SM, Brewer Jr HB, Cleeman JI, Smith Jr SC & Lenfant C (2004) Definition of metabolic syndrome: Report of the National Heart, Lung, and Blood Institute/American Heart Association conference on scientific issues related to definition. *Circulation* 109:433–8.

Isomaa B, Almgren P, Tuomi T, *et al.* (2001) Cardiovascular morbidity and mortality associated with the metabolic syndrome. *Diabetes Care* 24:683–9.

Jensen MD (2006) Is visceral fat involved in the pathogenesis of the metabolic syndrome? Human model. *Obesity (Silver Spring)* 14 (Suppl. 1):20S–24S.

Kylin E (1923) Studien uber das Hypertonie-Hyperglyka 'mie-Hyperurika' miesyndrom. *Zentralbl Inn Med* 44:105–127.

Lakka HM, Laaksonen DE, Lakka TA, *et al.* (2002) The metabolic syndrome and total and cardiovascular disease mortality in middle-aged men. *JAMA* 288:2709–16.

Lemieux I, Pascot A, Couillard C, *et al.* (2000) Hypertriglyceridemic waist: a marker of the atherogenic metabolic triad (hyperinsulinemia; hyperapolipoprotein B; small, dense LDL) in men? *Circulation* 102:179–84.

Meigs J (2003) The metabolic syndrome: may be a guidepost or detour to preventing type 2 diabetes and cardiovascular disease. *BMJ* 327:61–2.

Meigs JB, Wilson PW, Fox CS, *et al.* (2006) Body mass index, metabolic syndrome, and risk of type 2 diabetes or cardiovascular disease. *J Clin Endocrinol Metab* 91:2906–12.

Reaven GM (1988) Banting lecture 1988. Role of insulin resistance in human disease. *Diabetes* 37:1595–607.

Resnick HE (2002) Metabolic syndrome in American Indians. *Diabetes Care* 25:1246–7.

Sakkinen P, Wahl P, Cushman M, Lewis M & Tracy R (2000) Clustering of procoagulation, inflammation and fibrinolisis variables with metabolic factors in insulin resistance syndrome. *Am J Epidemiol* 152:897–907.

Weiss R, Dziura J, Burgert TS, *et al.* (2004) Obesity and the metabolic syndrome in children and adolescents. *N Engl J Med* 350:2362–74.

Adipose tissue as an endocrine organ

Barter P, McPherson YR, Song K, *et al.* (2007) Serum insulin and inflammatory markers in overweight individuals with and without dyslipidemia. *J Clin Endocrinol Metab* 92:2041–5.

Bastard JP, Maachi M, Lagathu C, *et al.* (2006) Recent advances in the relationship between obesity, inflammation, and insulin resistance. *Eur Cytokine Netw* 17:4–12.

Berg AH & Scherer PE (2005) Adipose tissue, inflammation, and cardiovascular disease. *Circ Res* 96; 939–49.

Bistrian BR & Khaodhiar L (2000) Chronic systemic inflammation in overweight and obese adults. *JAMA* 283:2235–6.

Fischer-Posovszky P, Wabitsch M & Hochberg Z (2007) Endocrinology of adipose tissue—an update. *Horm Metab Res* 39:314–21.

Fortuno A, Rodriguez A, Gomez-Ambrosi J, Fruhbeck G & Diez J (2003) Adipose tissue as an endocrine organ: role of leptin and adiponectin in the pathogenesis of cardiovascular diseases. *J Physiol Biochem* 59:51–60.

Frayn KN, Tan GD & Karpe F (2007) Adipose tissue: a key target for diabetes pathophysiology and treatment? *Horm Metab Res* 39:739–42.

Fruhbeck G (2004) The adipose tissue as a source of vasoactive factors. *Curr Med Chem Cardiovasc Hematol Agents* 2:197–208.

Guzik TJ, Mangalat D & Korbut R (2006) Adipocytokines—novel link between inflammation and vascular function? *J Physiol Pharmacol* 57:505–28.

Juge-Aubry CE, Henrichot E & Meier CA (2005) Adipose tissue: a regulator of inflammation. *Best Pract Res Clin Endocrinol Metab* 19; 547–66.

Kyrou I & Tsigos C (2007) Stress mechanisms and metabolic complications. *Horm Metab Res* 39:430–38.

Pou KM, Massaro JM, Hoffmann U, *et al.* (2007) Visceral and subcutaneous adipose tissue volumes are cross-sectionally related to markers of inflammation and oxidative stress: the Framingham Heart Study. *Circulation* 116:1234–41.

Rasouli N & Kern PA (2008) Adipocytokines and the metabolic complications of obesity. *J Clin Endocrinol Metab* 93 (Suppl. 1):S64–73.

Rodriguez A, Catalan V, Gomez-Ambrosi J & Fruhbeck G (2007) Visceral and subcutaneous adiposity: are both potential therapeutic targets for tackling the metabolic syndrome? *Curr Pharm Des* 13:2169–75.

Tilg H & Moschen AR (2006) Adipocytokines: mediators linking adipose tissue, inflammation and immunity. *Nat Rev Immunol* 6:772–83.

Trayhurn P & Wood IS (2004) Adipokines: inflammation and the pleiotropic role of white adipose tissue. *Brit J Nutr* 92:347–55.

Yudkin JS (2007) Inflammation, obesity, and the metabolic syndrome. *Horm Metab Res* 39:707–9.

Adiponectin

Date H, Imamura T, Ideguchi T, *et al.* (2006) Adiponectin produced in coronary circulation regulates coronary flow reserve in nondiabetic patients with angiographically normal coronary arteries. *Clin Cardiol* 29:211–4.

Eyileten Z, Yilmaz MI, Kaya K, *et al.* (2007) Coronary artery bypass grafting ameliorates the decreased plasma adiponectin level in atherosclerotic patients. *Tohoku J Exp Med* 213:71–7.

Iacobellis G, Tiziana di Gioia CR, Cotesta D, *et al.* (2008) Epicardial adipose tissue adiponectin expression is related to intracoronary adiponectin levels. *Horm Metab Res* 41:227–31.

Iacobellis G, Cotesta D, Petramala L, *et al.* (2009) Intracoronary adiponectin levels rapidly and significantly increase after coronary revascularization. *Int J Cardiol* (Epub ahead of print; doi:10.1016/j.ijcard.2008.12.155).

Kumada M, Kihara S, Sumitsuji S, *et al.* (2003) Association of hypoadiponectinemia with coronary artery disease in men. *Arterioscler Thromb Vasc Biol* 23:85–9.

Maahs DM, Ogden LG, Kinney GL, *et al.* (2005) Low plasma adiponectin levels predict progression of coronary artery calcification. *Circulation* 111:747–53.

Nakamura Y, Shimada K, Fukuda D, *et al.* (2004) Implications of plasma concentrations of adiponectin in patients with coronary artery disease. *Heart* 90:528–33.

Otsuka F, Sugiyama S, Kojima S, *et al.* (2006) Plasma adiponectin levels are associated with coronary lesion complexity in men with coronary artery disease. *J Am Coll Cardiol* 48:1155–62.

Ouchi N, Shibata R & Walsh K (2006) Cardioprotection by adiponectin. *Trends Cardiovasc Med* 16:141–6.

Pischon T, Girman CJ, Hotamisligil GS, Rifai N, Hu FB & Rimm EB (2004) Plasma adiponectin levels and risk of myocardial infarction in men. *JAMA* 291:1730–7.

Takano H, Kodama Y, Kitta Y, *et al.* (2006) Transcardiac adiponectin gradient is independently related to endothelial vasomotor function in large and resistance coronary arteries in humans. *Am J Physiol Heart Circ Physiol* 291:H2641–6.

Metabolically healthy obesity

Brochu M, Tchernof A & Dionne IJ (2001) What are the physical characteristics associated with a normal metabolic profile despite a high level of obesity in postmenopausal women? *J Clin Endocrinol Metab* 86:1020–5.

Iacobellis G, Ribaudo MC, Zappaterreno A & Leonetti F (2005) Prevalence of uncomplicated obesity in a Italian obese population. *Obes Res* 13:1116–22.

Karelis AD, St-Pierre DH, Conus F, Rabasa-Lhoret R & Poehlman ET (2004) Metabolic and body composition factors in subgroups of obesity: what do we know? *J Clin Endocrinol Metab* 89:2569–75.

Karelis AD, Faraj M, Bastard JP, *et al.* (2005) The metabolically healthy, but obese individual presents a favorable inflammation profile. *J Clin Endocrinol Metab* 90:4145–50.

Marchesini G, Melchionda N, Apolone G, *et al.* (2004) The metabolic syndrome in treatment-seeking obese persons. *Metabolism* 53:435–40.

Marini MA, Succurro E, Frontoni S, *et al.* (2007) Metabolically healthy but obese women have an intermediate cardiovascular risk profile between healthy non-obese women and obese insulin resistant women. *Diabetes Care* 30:2145–7.

Meigs JB, Wilson PW, Fox CS, *et al.* (2006) Body mass index, metabolic syndrome, and risk of type 2 diabetes or cardiovascular disease. *J Clin Endocrinol Metab* 91:2906–12.

Philip-Couderc P, Pathak A, Smih F, *et al.* (2004) Uncomplicated human obesity is associated with a specific cardiac transcriptome: involvement of the Wnt pathway. *FASEB J* 18:1539–40.

Shin MJ, Hyun YJ, Kim OY, Kim JY, Jang Y & Lee JH (2006) Weight loss effect on inflammation and LDL oxidation in metabolically healthy but obese (MHO) individuals: low inflammation and LDL oxidation in MHO women. *Int J Obes (Lond)* 30:1529–34.

Sims A (2001) Are there persons who are obese, but metabolically healthy? *Metabolism* 50:1499–504.

Wildman RP, Muntner P, Reynolds K, *et al.* (2008) The obese without cardiometabolic risk factorclustering and the normal weight with cardiometabolic risk factor clustering prevalence and correlates of 2 phenotypes among the US population (NHANES 1999–2004). *Arch Intern Med* 168:1617–24.

Obesity and the heart

Arias MA, Alonso-Fernandez A & Garcia-Rio F (2006) Left ventricular diastolic abnormalities in obese subjects. *Chest* 130:1282–3.

Barouch LA, Berkowitz DE, Harrison RW, O'Donnell CP & Hare JM (2003) Disruption of leptin signaling contributes to cardiac hypertrophy independently of body weight in mice. *Circulation* 108:754–9.

Crisostomo LL, Araujo LM, Camara E, *et al.* (1999) Comparison of left ventricular mass and function in obese versus nonobese women <40 years of age. *Am J Cardiol* 84:1127–9.

Daniels SR, Kimball TR, Morrison JA, Khoury P, Witt S & Meyer RA (1995) Effect of lean body mass, fat mass, blood pressure, and sexual maturation on left ventricular mass in children and adolescents: statistical, biological, and clinical significance. *Circulation* 92:3249–54.

DeFronzo RA, Cooke, CR, Andres R, Faloona GR & Davis PJ (1975) The effect of insulin on renal handling of sodium, potassium, calcium, and phosphate in man. *J Clin Invest* 55:845–55.

Delaughter MC, Taffet GE, Fiorotto ML, Entman ML & Schwartz RJ (1999) Local insulin-like growth factor I expression induces physiologic, then pathologic, cardiac hypertrophy in transgenic mice. *FASEB J* 13:1923–9.

Della Mea P, Lupia M, Bandolin V, *et al.* (2005) Adiponectin, insulin resistance, and left ventricular structure in dipper and nondipper essential hypertensive patients. *Am J Hypertens* 18:30–5.

Devereux RB, Alonso DR, Lutas EM, *et al.* (1986) Echocardiographic assessment of left ventricular hypertrophy: comparison to necropsy findings. *Am J Cardiol* 57:450–8.

Dorbala S, Crugnale S, Yang D & Di Carli MF (2006) Effect of body mass index on left ventricular cavity size and ejection fraction. *Am J Cardiol* 97:725–9.

Galvan AQ, Galetta F, Natali A, *et al.* (2000) Insulin resistance and hyperinsulinemia: no independent relation to left ventricular mass in humans. *Circulation* 102:2233–8.

Gomez-Ambrosi J, Salvador J, Silva C, *et al.* (2006) Increased cardiovascular risk markers in obesity are associated with body adiposity: role of leptin. *Thromb Haemost* 95:991–6.

Grandi AM, Zanzi P, Fachinetti A, *et al.* (1999) Insulin and diastolic dysfunction in lean and obese hypertensives. *Hypertension* 34:1208–14.

Greenwood JP, Scott EM, Stoker JB & Mary DA (2001) Hypertensive left ventricular hypertrophy: relation to peripheral sympathetic drive. *J Am Coll Cardiol* 15:1711–17.

Hong SJ, Park CG, Seo HS, Oh DJ & Ro YM (2004) Associations among plasma adiponectin, hypertension, left ventricular diastolic function and left ventricular mass index. *Blood Press* 13:236–42.

Iacobellis G (2004) True uncomplicated obesity is not related to increased left ventricular mass and systolic dysfunction. *J Am Coll Cardiol* 44:2257.

Iacobellis G & Sharma AM (2007) Obesity and the heart: redefinition of the relationship. *Obes Rev* 8:35–9.

Iacobellis G, Ribaudo MC, Leto G, *et al.* (2002) Influence of excess fat on cardiac morphology and function: study in uncomplicated obesity. *Obes Res* 10:767–73.

Iacobellis G, Ribaudo MC, Zappaterreno A, Vecci E, Di Mario U & Leonetti F (2003) Relationship of insulin sensitivity and left ventricular mass in uncomplicated obesity. *Obes Res* 11:518–24.

Iacobellis G, Petrone A, Leonetti F & Buzzetti R (2006) Left ventricular mass and +276G/G single nucleotide polymorphism of the adiponectin gene in uncomplicated obesity. *Obesity (Silver Spring)* 14:368–72.

Iacobellis G, Ribaudo MC, Zappaterreno A, Iannucci CV, Di Mario U & Leonetti F (2004) Adapted changes in left ventricular structure and function in severe uncomplicated obesity. *Obes Res* 12:1616–21.

Iacobellis G, Pond CM & Sharma AM (2006) Different 'weight' of cardiac and general adiposity in predicting left ventricle morphology obesity. 14:1679–84.

Jain A, Avendano G, Dharamsey S, *et al.* (1996) Left ventricular diastolic function in hypertension and role of plasma glucose and insulin: comparison with diabetic heart. *Circulation* 93:1396–1402.

Kamide K, Rakugi H, Higaki J, *et al.* (2002) The renin–angiotensin and adrenergic nervous system in cardiac hypertrophy in fructose-fed rats. *Am J Hypertens* 15:66–71.

Krishnan R, Becker RJ, Beighley LM & Lopez-Candales A (2005) Impact of body mass index on markers of left ventricular thickness and mass calculation: results of a pilot analysis. *Echocardiography* 22:203–10.

Malmqvist K, Isaksson H, Ostergren J & Kahan T (2001) Left ventricular mass is not related to insulin sensitivity in never-treated primary hypertension. *J Hypertens* 19:311–17.

Malmqvist K, Ohman KP, Lind L, Nystrom F & Kahan T (2002) Relationships between left ventricular mass and the renin–angiotensin system, catecholamines, insulin and leptin. *J Intern Med* 252:430–9.

Mitsuhashi H, Yatsuya H, Tamakoshi K, *et al.* (2007) Adiponectin level and left ventricular hypertrophy in Japanese men. *Hypertension* 49:1448–54.

Mureddu GF, de Simone G, Greco R, Rosato GF & Contaldo F (1996) Left ventricular filling pattern in uncomplicated obesity. *Am J Cardiol* 77:509–14.

Mureddu GF, Greco R, Rosato GF, *et al.* (1998) Relation of insulin resistance to left ventricular hypertrophy and diastolic dysfunction in obesity. *Int J Obes Relat Metab Disord* 22:363–8.

Otto ME, Belohlavek M, Khandheria B, Gilman G, Svatikova A & Somers V (2004) Comparison of right and left ventricular function in obese and nonobese men. *Am J Cardiol* 93:1569–72.

Paolisso G, Manzella D, Montano N, Gambardella A & Varricchio M (2000) Plasma leptin concentrations and cardiac autonomic nervous system in healthy subjects with different body weights. *J Clin Endocrinol Metab* 85,1810–14.

Paolisso G, Tagliamonte MR, Galderisi M, *et al.* (2001) Plasma leptin concentration, insulin sensitivity, and 24-hour ambulatory blood pressure and left ventricular geometry. *Am J Hypertens* 14:114–20.

Pascual M, Pascual DA, Soria F, *et al.* (2003) Effects of isolated obesity on systolic and diastolic left ventricular function. *Heart* 89:1152–6.

Peterson LR, Waggoner AD, Schechtman KB, *et al.* (2004) Alterations in left ventricular structure and function in young healthy obese women: assessment by echocardiography and tissue Doppler imaging. *J Am Coll Cardiol* 43:1399–404.

Pladevall M, Williams K, Guyer H, *et al.* (2003) The association between leptin and left ventricular hypertrophy: a population-based cross-sectional study. *J Hypertens* 21:1467–73.

Powell BD, Redfield MM, Bybee KA, Freeman WK & Rihal CS (2006) Association of obesity with left ventricular remodeling and diastolic dysfunction in patients without coronary artery disease. *Am J Cardiol* 98:116–20.

Sader S, Nian M & Liu P (2003) Leptin: a novel link between obesity, diabetes, cardiovascular risk, and ventricular hypertrophy. *Circulation* 108:644–6.

Sasson Z, Rasooly Y, Gupta R & Rasooly I (1996) Left atrial enlargement in healthy obese: prevalence and relation to left ventricular mass and diastolic function. *Can J Cardiol* 12:257–263.

Sundström J, Lind L, Nyström N, *et al.* (2000) Left ventricular concentric remodeling rather than left ventricular hypertrophy is related to the insulin resistance syndrome in elderly men. *Circulation* 101:2595–600.

Tanaka N, Ryoke T, Hongo M, *et al.* (1998) Effects of growth hormone and IGF-I on cardiac hypertrophy and gene expression in mice. *Am J Physiol* 275:H393–99.

Tritos NA, Manning WJ & Danias PG (2004) Role of leptin in the development of cardiac hypertrophy in experimental animals and humans. *Circulation* 109:e67.

Valencia-Flores M, Rebollar V, Santiago V, *et al.* (2004) Prevalence of pulmonary hypertension and its association with respiratory disturbances in obese patients living at moderately high altitude. *Int J Obes Relat Metab Disord* 28:1174–80.

Watanabe K, Sekiya M, Tsuruoka T, Funada J & Kameoka H (1999) Effect of insulin resistance on left ventricular hypertrophy and dysfunction in essential hypertension. *J Hypertens* 17:1153–60.

Wong CY, O'Moore-Sullivan T, Leano R, Byrne N, Beller E & Marwick TH (2004) Alterations of left ventricular myocardial characteristics associated with obesity. *Circulation* 110:3081–7.

Epicardial adipose tissue

Ahn SG, Lim HS, Joe DY, *et al.* (2008) Relationship of epicardial adipose tissue by echocardiography to coronary artery disease. *Heart* 94:e7.

Baker AR, Silva NF, Quinn DW, *et al.* (2006) Human epicardial adipose tissue expresses a pathogenic profile of adipocytokines in patients with cardiovascular disease. *Cardiovasc Diabetol* 5:1–7.

Chaldakov GN, Fiore M, Stankulov IS, *et al.* (2004) Neurotrophin presence in human coronary atherosclerosis and metabolic syndrome: a role for NGF and BDNF in cardiovascular disease? *Prog Brain Res* 146:279–89.

Chaowalit N, Somers VK, Pellikka PA, Rihal CS &Lopez-Jimenez F (2006) Subepicardial adipose tissue and the presence and severity of coronary artery disease. *Atherosclerosis* 186:354–9.

Cheng KH, Chu CS, Lee KT, *et al.* (2008) Adipocytokines and proinflammatory mediators from abdominal and epicardial adipose tissue in patients with coronary artery disease. *Int J Obes (Lond)* 32:268–74.

Corradi D, Maestri R, Callegari S, *et al.* (2004) The ventricular epicardial fat is related to the myocardial mass in normal, ischemic and hypertrophic hearts. *Cardiovasc Pathol* 13:313–16.

de Vos AM, Prokop M, Roos CJ, *et al.* (2007) Peri-coronary epicardial adipose tissue is related to cardiovascular risk factors and coronary artery calcification in post-menopausal women. *Eur Heart J* 29:777–83.

Ding J, Kritchevsky SB, Harris TB, *et al.* (2008) The association of pericardial fat with calcified coronary plaque. *Obesity* 16:1914–9.

Fain JN, Sacks HS, Buehrer B, *et al.* (2008) Identification of omentin mRNA in human epicardial adipose tissue: comparison to omentin in subcutaneous, internal mammary artery periadventitial and visceral abdominal depots. *Int J Obes (Lond)* 32:810–5.

Iacobellis G (2006) Adiposity of the heart. *Ann Intern Med* 145:554–5.

Iacobellis G & Barbaro G (2008) The double role of epicardial adipose tissue as pro- and anti-inflammatory organ. *Horm Metab Res* 40:442–5.

Iacobellis G & Leonetti F (2005) Epicardial adipose tissue and insulin resistance in obese subjects. *J Clin Endocrinol Metab* 90:6300–2.

Iacobellis G & Sharma AM (2007) Epicardial adipose tissue as new cardio-metabolic risk marker and potential therapeutic target in the metabolic syndrome. *Curr Pharm Des* 13:2180–4.

Iacobellis G, Assael F, Ribaudo MC, *et al.* (2003) Epicardial fat from echocardiography: a new method for visceral adipose tissue prediction. *Obes Res* 11:304–10.

Iacobellis G, Ribaudo MC, Assael F, *et al.* (2003) Echocardiographic epicardial adipose tissue is related to anthropometric and clinical parameters of metabolic syndrome: a new indicator of cardiovascular risk. *J Clin Endocrinol Metab* 88:5163–8.

Iacobellis G, Ribaudo MC, Zappaterreno A, Iannucci CV & Leonetti F (2004) Relation between epicardial adipose tissue and left ventricular mass. *Am J Cardiol* 94:1084–7.

Iacobellis G, Corradi D & Sharma AM (2005) Epicardial adipose tissue: anatomic, biomolecular and clinical relationships with the heart. *Nat Clin Pract Cardiovasc Med* 2:536–43.

Iacobellis G, Pistilli D, Gucciardo M, *et al.* (2005) Adiponectin expression in human epicardial adipose tissue in vivo is lower in patients with coronary artery disease. *Cytokine* 29:251–5.

Iacobellis G, Leonetti F, Singh N, Sharma AM (2007) Relationship of epicardial adipose tissue with atrial dimensions and diastolic function in morbidly obese subjects. *Int J Cardiol* 115:272–3.

Iacobellis G, Pellicelli AM, Sharma AM, Grisorio B, Barbarini G & Barbaro G (2007) Relation of subepicardial adipose tissue to carotid intima-media thickness in patients with human immunodeficiency virus. *Am J Cardiol* 99:1470–2.

Iacobellis G, Barbaro G & Gerstein HC (2008) Relationship of epicardial fat thickness and fasting glucose. *Int J Cardiol* 128:424–6.

Iacobellis G, Gao YJ & Sharma AM (2008) Do cardiac and perivascular adipose tissue play a role in atherosclerosis? *Curr Diab Rep* 8:20–4.

Iacobellis G, Pellicelli AM, Grisorio B, *et al.* (2008) Relation of epicardial fat and alanine aminotransferase in subjects with increased visceral fat. *Obesity* 16:179–83.

Iacobellis G, Singh N, Wharton S & Sharma AM (2008) Substantial changes in epicardial fat thickness after weight loss in severely obese subjects. *Obesity* 16:1693–7.

Iacobellis G, Willens HJ, Barbaro G & Sharma AM (2008) Threshold values of high-risk echocardiographic epicardial fat thickness. *Obesity* 16:887–92.

Jeong JW, Jeong MH, Yun KH, *et al.* (2007) Echocardiographic epicardial fat thickness and coronary artery disease. *Circ J* 71:536–9.

Kankaanpaa M, Lehto HR, Parkka J, *et al.* (2006) Myocardial triglyceride content and epicardial fat mass in human obesity: relationship to left ventricular function and serum free fatty acid levels. *J Clin Endocrinol Metab* 91:4689–95.

Kremen J, Dolinkova M, Krajickova J, *et al.* (2006) Increased subcutaneous and epicardial adipose tissue production of proinflammatory cytokines in cardiac surgery patients: possible role in postoperative insulin resistance. *J Clin Endocrinol Metab* 46:20–7.

Lanes R, Soros A, Flores K Gunczler P, Carrillo E & Bandel J (2005) Endothelial function, carotid artery intima-media thickness, epicardial adipose tissue, and left ventricular mass and function in growth hormone-deficient adolescents: apparent effects of growth hormone treatment on these parameters. *J Clin Endocrinol Metab* 90:3978–82.

Malavazos AE, Ermetici F, Cereda E, *et al.* (2007) Epicardial fat thickness: relationship with plasma visfatin and plasminogen activator inhibitor-1 levels in visceral obesity. *Nutr Metab Cardiovasc Dis* 18:523–30.

Malavazos AE, Ermetici F, Coman C, Corsi MM, Morricone L & Ambrosi B (2007) Influence of epicardial adipose tissue and adipocytokine levels on cardiac abnormalities in visceral obesity. *Int J Cardiol* 121:132–4.

Marchington JM & Pond CM (1990) Site specific properties of pericardial and epicardial adipose tissue: the effects of insulin and high-fat feeding on lipogenesis and the incorporation of fatty acids in vivo. *Int J Obesity* 14:1013–22.

Mazurek T, Zhang L, Zalewski A, *et al.* (2003) Human epicardial adipose tissue is a source of inflammatory mediators. *Circulation* 108:2460–6.

Rabkin RW (2007) Epicardial fat: properties, function and relationship to obesity. *Obes Rev* 8:253–61.

Reiner L, Mazzoleni A & Rodriguez FL (1955) Statistical analysis of the epicardial fat weight in human hearts. *AMA Arch Pathol* 60:369–73.

Sacks HS & Fain JN (2007) Human epicardial adipose tissue: a review. *Am Heart J* 153:907–17.

Schejbal V (1989) Epicardial fatty tissue of the right ventricle: morphology, morphometry and functional significance. *Pneumologie* 43:490–9 (in German).

Silaghi A, Achard V, Paulmyer-Lacroix O, *et al.* (2007) Expression of adrenomedullin in human epicardial adipose tissue: role of coronary status. *Am J Physiol Endocrinol Metab* 293:E1443–50.

Perivascular adipose tissue

Barandier C, Montani JP & Yang Z (2005) Mature adipocytes and perivascular adipose tissue stimulate vascular smooth muscle cell proliferation: effects of aging and obesity. *Am J Physiol Heart Circ Physiol* 289:H1807–13.

Dubrovska G, Verlohren S, Luft FC & Gollasch M (2004) Mechanisms of ADRF release from rat aortic adventitial adipose tissue. *Am J Physiol* 286:H1107–13.

Engeli S (2005) Is there a pathophysiological role for perivascular adipocytes? *Am J Physiol Heart Circ Physiol* 289:H1794–5.

Frühbeck G (1999) Pivotal role of nitric oxide in the control of blood pressure after leptin administration. *Diabetes* 48:903–8.

Galvez B, de Castro J, Herold D, *et al.* (2006) Perivascular adipose tissue and mesenteric vascular function in spontaneously hypertensive rats. *Arterioscler Thromb Vasc Biol* 26:1297–302.

Gao YJ, Zeng ZH, Teoh K, *et al.* (2005) Perivascular adipose tissue modulates vascular function in the human internal thoracic artery. *J Thorac Cardiovasc Surg* 130:1130–6.

Gao YJ, Takemori K, Su LY, *et al.* (2006) Perivascular adipose tissue promotes vasoconstriction: the role of superoxide anion. *Cardiovasc Res* 71:363–73.

Gollasch M & Dubrovska G (2004) Paracrine role for periadventitial adipose tissue in the regulation of arterial tone. *Trends Pharmacol Sci* 25:647–53.

Henrichot E, Juge-Aubry CE, Pernin A, *et al.* (2005) Production of chemokines by perivascular adipose tissue: a role in the pathogenesis of atherosclerosis? *Arterioscler Thromb Vasc Biol* 25:2594–9.

Löhn M, Dubrovska G, Lauterbach B, Luft FC, Gollasch M & Sharma AM (2002) Periadventitial fat releases a vascular relaxing factor. *FASEB J* 16:1057–63.

Montani JP, Carroll JF, Dwyer TM, Antic V, Yang Z & Dulloo AG (2004) Ectopic fat storage in heart, blood vessels and kidneys in the pathogenesis of cardiovascular diseases. *Int J Obes Relat Metab Disord* 28 (Suppl. 4):S58–65.

Soltis EE & Cassis LA (1991) Influence of perivascular adipose tissue on rat aortic smooth muscle responsiveness. *Clin Exp Hypertens* 275:681–92.

Verlohren, Dubrovska G, Tsang S-Y, *et al.* (2004) Visceral periadventitial adipose tissue regulates arterial tone of mesenteric arteries. *Hypertension* 44:271–26.

Intra-myocardial fat

Chiu HC, Kovacs A, Ford DA, *et al.* (2001) A novel mouse model of lipotoxic cardiomyopathy. *J Clin Invest* 107:813–22.

Iacobellis G & Sharma AM (2006) Adiposity of the heart. *Ann Intern Med* 145:554–5.

McGavock JM, Victor RG, Unger RH & Szczepaniak LS (2006) Adiposity of the heart, revisited. *Ann Intern Med* 144:517–24.

Reingold JS, McGavock JM, Kaka S, Tillery T, Victor RG & Szczepaniak LS (2005) Determination of triglyceride in the human myocardium using magnetic resonance spectroscopy: reproducibility and sensitivity of the method. *Am J Physiol Endocrinol Metab* 289:E935–9.

Szczepaniak LS, Dobbins RL, Metzger GJ, *et al.* (2003) Myocardial triglycerides and systolic function in humans: in vivo evaluation by localized proton spectroscopy and cardiac imaging. *Magn Reson Med* 49:417–23.

Zhou YT, Grayburn P, Karim A, *et al.* (2000) Lipotoxic heart disease in obese rats: implications for human obesity. *Proc Natl Acad Sci USA* 97:1784–9.

Anthropometric indices of adiposity.

Ajani UA, Lotufo PA, Gaziano JM, *et al.* (2004) Body mass index and mortality among US male physicians. *Ann Epidemiol* 14:731–9.

Dagenais GR, Yi Q, Mann JF, Bosch J, Pogue J & Yusuf S (2005) Prognostic impact of body weight and abdominal obesity in women and men with cardiovascular disease. *Am Heart J* 159:54–60.

de Koning L, Merchant AT, Pogue J & Anand SS (2007) Waist circumference and waist-to-hip ratio as predictors of cardiovascular events: meta-regression analysis of prospective studies. *Eur Heart J* 28:850–6.

Janssen I, Katzmarzyk PT & Ross R (2004) Waist circumference and not body mass index explains obesity-related health risk. *Am J Clin Nutr* 79:379–84.

Janssen I, Katzmarzyk PT & Ross R (2005) Body mass index is inversely related to mortality in older people after adjustment for waist circumference. *J Am Geriatr Soc* 53:2112–8.

Jensen MD (2008) Role of body fat distribution and the metabolic complications of obesity. *J Clin Endocrinol Metab* 93 (Suppl. 1):S57–63.

Kuk JL, Janiszewski PM & Ross R (2007) Body mass index and hip and thigh circumferences are negatively associated with visceral adipose tissue after control for waist circumference. *Am J Clin Nutr* 85:1540–4.

Rexrode KM, Carey VJ, Hennekens CH, Walters EE, Colditz GA, Stampfer MJ, Willett WC, Manson JE (1998) Abdominal adiposity and coronary heart disease in women. *JAMA* 280:1843–8.

Widlansky ME, Sesso HD, Rexrode KM, Manson JE, Gaziano JM (2004) Body mass index and total and cardiovascular mortality in men with a history of cardiovascular disease. *Arch Intern Med* 164:2326–32.

Zhang X, Shu XO, Gao YT, *et al.* (2004) Anthropometric predictors of coronary heart disease in Chinese women. *Int J Obes Relat Metab Disord* 28:734–40.

Imaging of adiposity

Abbara S, Desai JC, Ricardo CC, Butler J, Nieman K & Reddy V (2005) Mapping epicardial fat with multidetector computed tomography to facilitate percutaneous transepicardial arrhythmia ablation. *Eur J Radiol* 57:417–22.

Abe T, Kawakami Y, Sugita M, *et al.* (1991) Sonography detection of small intra-abdominal fat variations. *Int J Obes* 15:847–52.

Abe T, Kawakami Y, Sugita M, Yoshikawa K & Fukunaga T (1995) Use of B-mode ultrasound for visceral fat mass evaluation: comparisons with magnetic resonance imaging. *Appl Human Sci* 14:133–9.

Armellini F, Zamboni M, Rigo L, *et al.* (1990) The contribution of sonography to the measurement of intra-abdominal fat. *J Clin Ultrasound* 18:563–7.

Armellini, F, Zamboni, M, Robbi, R, *et al.* (1993) Total and intra-abdominal fat measurements by ultrasound and computerized tomography. *Int J Obes Relat Metab Disord* 17:209–14.

Ferrozzi, F, Zuccoli, G, Tognini, G, *et al.* (1999) An assessment of abdominal fatty tissue distribution in obese children. A comparison between echography and computed tomography. *Radiol Med (Torino)* 98:490–4 (in Italian).

Fluchter S, Haghi D, Dinter D, *et al.* (2007) Volumetric assessment of epicardial adipose tissue with cardiovascular magnetic resonance imaging. *Obesity* 15:870–8.

Goodpaster BH (2002) Measuring body fat distribution and content in humans. *Curr Opin Clin Nutr Metab Care* 5:481–7.

Iacobellis G (2005) Imaging of visceral adipose tissue: an emerging diagnostic tool and therapeutic target. *Curr Drug Targets Cardiovasc Haematol Disord* 5:345–53.

Kawamoto R, Kajiwara T, Oka Y & Takagi Y (2002) Association between abdominal wall fat index and carotid atherosclerosis in women. *J Atheroscler Thromb* 9:213–8.

Kim K, Kim HJ, Hur KY, *et al.* (2004) Visceral fat thickness measured by ultrasonography can estimate not only visceral obesity but also risks of cardiovascular and metabolic diseases. *Am J Clinical Nutrition* 79:593–9.

Koester RS, Hunter GR, Snyder S, Khaled MA & Berland LL (1992) Estimation of computerized tomography derived abdominal fat distribution. *Int J Obes Relat Metab Disord* 16:543–54.

Kvist H, Chowdhury B, Grangard U, Tylén U & Sjöström L (1988) Total and visceral adipose-tissue volumes derived from measurements with computed tomography in adult men and women: predictive equations. *Am J Clin Nutr* 48:1351–61.

Leite CC, Wajchenberg BL, Radominski R, Matsuda D, Cerri GG & Halpern A (2002) Intra-abdominal thickness by ultrasonography to predict risk factors for cardiovascular disease and its correlation with anthropometric measurements. *Metabolism* 51:1034–40.

Liu KH, Chan YL, Chan WB, Kong WL, Kong MO & Chan JC (2003) Sonographic measurement of mesenteric fat thickness is a good correlate with cardiovascular risk factors: comparison with subcutaneous and preperitoneal fat thickness, magnetic resonance imaging and anthropometric indexes. *Int J Obes Relat Metab Disord* 27:1267–73.

Suzuki R, Watanabe S, Hirai Y, *et al.* (1993) Abdominal wall fat index, estimated by ultrasonography, for assessment of the ratio of visceral fat to subcutaneous fat in the abdomen. *Am J Med* 95:309–14.

Ribeiro-Filho FF, Faria AN, Kohlmann O (2001) Ultrasonography for the evaluation of visceral fat and cardiovascular risk. *Hypertension* 38, 713–7.

Ribeiro-Filho FF, Faria AN, Azjen S, Zanella MT & Ferreira SR (2003) Methods of estimation of visceral fat: advantages of ultrasonography. *Obes Res* 11:1488–94.

Ross R (2003) Advances in the application of imaging methods in applied and clinical physiology. *Acta Diabetol* 40 (Suppl. 1):S45–50.

Ross RL, Leger D, Morris D, de Guise J & Guardo R (1992) Quantification of adipose tissue by MRI: relationship with anthropometric variables. *J Appl Physiol* 72:787–95.

Ross R, Shaw KD, Martel Y, de Guise J & Avruch L (1993) Adipose tissue distribution measured by magnetic resonance imaging in obese women. *Am J Clin Nutr* 57:470–5.

Ross R, Shaw KD, Martel Y, de Guise J, Hudson R & Avruch L (1993) Determination of total and regional adipose tissue distribution by magnetic resonance imaging in android women. *Basic Life Sci* 60:177–80.

Ross R, Shaw KD, Rissanen J, Martel Y, de Guise J & Avruch L (1994) Sex differences in lean and adipose tissue distribution by magnetic resonance imaging: anthropometric relationships. *Am J Clin Nutr* 59:1277–85.

Ross R, Goodpaster B, Kelley D & Boada F (2000) Magnetic resonance imaging in human body composition research. From quantitative to qualitative tissue measurement. *Ann N Y Acad Sci* 904:12–7.

Schoen RE, Evans RW, Sankey SS, Weissfeld JL & Kuller L (1996) Does visceral adipose tissue differ from subcutaneous adipose tissue in fatty acid content? *Int J Obes Relat Metab Disord* 20:346–52.

Shen W, Wang Z, Punyanita M, *et al.* (2003) Adipose tissue quantification by imaging methods: a proposed classification. *Obes Res* 11:5–16.

Stolk RP, Meijer R, Mali WP, Grobbee DE & van der Graaf Y (2003) Ultrasound measurements of intraabdominal fat estimate the metabolic syndrome better than do measurements of waist circumference. *Am J Clin Nutr* 77:857–60.

Stolk RP, Wink O, Zelissen PM, Meijer R, van Gils AP & Grobbee DE (2001) Validity and reproducibility of ultrasonography for the measurement of intra-abdominal adipose tissue. *Int J Obes Relat Metab Disord* 25:1346–51.

Straeter-Knowlen IM, Evanochko WT, den Hollander JA, *et al.* (1996) ^{1}H NMR spectroscopic imaging of myocardial triglycerides in excised dog hearts subjected to 24 hours of coronary occlusion. *Circulation* 93:1464–70.

Szczepaniak LS, Babcock EE, Schick F, *et al.* (1999) Measurement of intracellular triglyceride stores by H spectroscopy: validation in vivo. *Am J Physiol* 276:E977–89.

Tayama K, Inukai T & Shimomura Y (1999) Preperitoneal fat deposition estimated by ultrasonography in patients with non-insulin-dependent diabetes mellitus. *Diabetes Res Clin Pract* 43:49–58.

Thomas EL, Saeed N, Hajnal JV, *et al.* (1998) Magnetic resonance imaging of total body fat. *J Appl Physiol* 85:1778–85.

Vague J & Fenasse R (1965) Comparative anatomy of adipose tissue. In *Adipose Tissue*, edited by AE Renold & GF Cahill, pp. 25–36. Washington, DC: American Physiological Society.

Zhou YT, Grayburn P, Karim A, *et al.* (2000) Lipotoxic heart disease in obese rats: implications for human obesity. *Proc Natl Acad Sci U S A* 97:1784–9.

Obesity and hypertension

Aucott L, Poobalan A, Smith WC, Avenell A, Jung R & Broom J (2005) Effects of weight loss in overweight/obese individuals and long-term hypertension outcomes: a systematic review. *Hypertension* 45:1035–41.

Dentali F, Sharma AM & Douketis JD (2005) Management of hypertension in overweight and obese patients: a practical guide for clinicians. *Curr Hypertens Rep* 7:330–6.

Droyvold WB, Midthjell K, Nilsen TI & Holmen J (2005) Change in body mass index and its impact on blood pressure: a prospective population study. *Int J Obes (Lond)* 29:650–5.

Kurukulasuriya LR, Stas S, Lastra G, Manrique C & Sowers JR (2008) Hypertension in obesity. *Endocrinol Metab Clin North Am* 37:647–62.

Lin S, Cheng TO, Liu X, *et al.* (2006) Impact of dysglycemia, body mass index, and waist-to-hip ratio on the prevalence of systemic hypertension in a lean Chinese population. *Am J Cardiol* 97:839–42.

Schmieder RE & Messerli FH (1993) Does obesity influence early target organ damage in hypertensive patients? *Circulation* 87:1482–8.

Sharma AM (2004) Is there a rationale for angiotensin blockade in the management of obesity hypertension? *Hypertension* 44:12–19.

Sharma AM (2004) Mediastinal fat, insulin resistance, and hypertension. *Hypertension* 44:117–8.

Sharma AM & Chetty VT (2005) Obesity, hypertension and insulin resistance. *Acta Diabetol* 42 (Suppl. 1):S3–8.

Sharma AM, Pischon T, Engeli S, Scholze J (2001) Choice of drug treatment for obesity-related hypertension: where is the evidence? *J Hypertens* 19:667–74.

Sharma AM, Janke J, Gorzelniak K, Engeli S & Luft FC (2002) Angiotensin blockade prevents type 2 diabetes by formation of fat cells. *Hypertension* 40:609–11.

Wassertheil-Smoller S, Fann C, Allman RM, *et al.* (2000) Relation of low body mass to death and stroke in the systolic hypertension in the elderly program. The SHEP Cooperative Research Group. *Arch Intern Med* 160:494–500.

The obesity paradox

Curtis JP, Selter JG, Wang Y, *et al.* (2005) The obesity paradox: body mass index and outcomes in patients with heart failure. *Arch Intern Med* 165:55–61.

Davos H, Doehner W, Rauchhaus M, *et al.* (2003) Body mass and survival in patients with chronic heart failure without cachexia: the importance of obesity. *J Card Fail* 9:29–35.

Fonarow GC, Srikanthan P, Costanzo MR, Cintron GB, Lopatin M & the ADHERE Scientific Advisory Committee and Investigators (2007) An obesity paradox in acute heart failure: analysis of body mass index and inhospital mortality for 108,927 patients in the Acute Decompensated Heart Failure National Registry. *Am Heart J* 153:74–81.

Gustafsson F, Kragelund CB, Torp-Pedersen C, *et al.* (2005) Effect of obesity and being overweight on long-term mortality in congestive heart failure: influence of left ventricular systolic function. *Eur Heart J* 26:58–64.

Habbu A, Lakkis NM & Dokainish H (2006) The obesity paradox: fact or fiction? *Am J Cardiol* 98:944–8.

Horwich TB, Fonarow GC, Hamilton MA, MacLellan WR, Woo MA & Tillisch JH (2001) The relationship between obesity and mortality in patients with heart failure. *J Am Coll Cardiol* 38:789–95.

Lissin LW, Gauri AJ, Froelicher VF, Ghayoumi A, Myers J, & Giacommini J (2002) The prognostic value of body mass index and standard exercise testing in male veterans with congestive heart failure. *J Card Fail* 8:206–15.

Mariotti R, Castrogiovanni F, Becherini F, Cortese B, Rondinini L & Mariani M (2004) Obesity, weight loss and heart failure. *Eur Heart J Suppl* 6 (Suppl. F): F87–90.

Oreopoulos A, Padwal R, Kalantar-Zadeh K, Fonarow GC, Norris CM & McAlister FA (2008) Body mass index and mortality in heart failure: a meta-analysis. *Am Heart J* 156:13–22.

Obesity and coronary artery disease

Brandt M, Harder K, Walluscheck KP, *et al.* (2001) Severe obesity does not adversely affect perioperative mortality and morbidity in coronary artery bypass surgery. *Eur J Cardiothorac Surg* 19:662–6.

Diercks DB, Roe MT, Mulgund J, *et al.* (2006) The obesity paradox in non-ST-segment elevation acute coronary syndromes: results from the Can Rapid risk stratification of Unstable angina patients Suppress ADverse outcomes with Early implementation of the American College of Cardiology/American Heart Association Guidelines Quality Improvement Initiative. *Am Heart J* 152:140–8.

Domanski MJ, Jablonski KA, Rice MM, Fowler SE, Braunwald E & the PEACE Investigators (2006) Obesity and cardiovascular events in patients with established coronary disease. *Eur Heart J* 27:1416–22.

Gurm HS, Whitlow PL, Kip KE & the BARI Investigators (2002) The impact of body mass index on short- and long-term outcomes inpatients undergoing coronary revascularization. Insights from the bypass angioplasty revascularization investigation (BARI). *J Am Coll Cardiol* 39:834–40.

Hoit BD, Gilpin EA, Maisel AA, Henning H, Carlisle J & Ross J (1987) Influence of obesity on morbidity and mortality after acute myocardial infarction. *Am Heart J* 114:1334–41.

Hubert HB, Feinleib M, McNamara PM & Castelli WP (1983) Obesity as an independent risk factor for cardiovascular disease: a 26-year follow-up of the participants in the Framingham Heart Study. *Circulation* 67:968–77.

Kaplan RC, Heckbert SR, Furberg CD & Psaty BM (2002) Predictors of subsequent coronary events, stroke, and death among survivors of first hospitalized myocardial infarction. *J Clin Epidemiol* 55:654–64.

Kim J, Hammar N, Jakobsson K, Luepker RV, McGovern PG & Ivert T (2003) Obesity and the risk of early and late mortality after coronary artery bypass graft surgery. *Am Heart J* 146:555–60.

Minutello RM, Chou ET, Hong MK, *et al.* (2004) Impact of body mass index on in-hospital outcomes following percutaneous coronary intervention (report from the New York State Angioplasty Registry). *Am J Cardiol* 93:1229–32.

Rabkin SW, Mathewson FA & Hsu PH (1977) Relation of body weight to development of ischemic heart disease in a cohort of young North American men after a 26 year observation period: the Manitoba Study. *Am J Cardiol* 39:452–8.

Rana JS, Mukamal KJ, Morgan JP, Muller JE & Mittleman MA (2004) Obesity and the risk of death after acute myocardial infarction. *Am Heart J* 147:841–6.

Rea TD, Heckbert SR, Kaplan RC, *et al.* (2001) Body mass index and the risk of recurrent coronary events following acute myocardial infarction. *Am J Cardiol* 88:467–72.

Reeves BC, Ascione R, Chamberlain MH & Angelini GD (2003) Effect of body mass index on early outcomes in patients undergoing coronary artery bypass surgery. *J Am Coll Cardiol* 42:668–76.

Romero-Corral A, Montori VM, Somers VK, *et al.* (2006) Association of bodyweight with total mortality and with cardiovascular events in coronary artery disease: a systematic review of cohort studies. *Lancet* 368:666–78.

Todd Miller M, Lavie CJ & White CJ (2008) Impact of obesity on the pathogenesis and prognosis of coronary heart disease. *J Cardiometab Syndr* 3:162–7.

Wilson PW, D'Agostino RB, Sullivan L, Parise H & Kannel WB (2002) Overweight and obesity as determinants of cardiovascular risk: the Framingham experience. *Arch Intern Med* 162:1867–72.

Obesity and arrhythmias

Alpert MA, Terry BE, Cohen MV, Fan TM, Painter JA & Massey CV (2000) The electrocardiogram in morbid obesity. *Am J Cardiol* 85:908–10.

Brown DW, Giles WH, Greenlund KJ, Valdez R & Croft JB (2001) Impaired fasting glucose, diabetes mellitus, and cardiovascular disease risk factors are associated with prolonged QTc duration: results from the Third National Health and Nutrition Examination Survey. *J Cardiovasc Risk* 8:227–33.

Dublin S, French B, Glazer NL, *et al.* (2006) Risk of new-onset atrial fibrillation in relation to body mass index. *Arch Intern Med* 166:2322–8.

el-Gamal A, Gallagher D, Nawras A, *et al.* (1995) Effects of obesity on QT, RR, and QTc intervals. *Am J Cardiol* 75:956–9.

Gami AS, Hodge DO, Herges RM, *et al.* (2007) Obstructive sleep apnea, obesity, and the risk of incident atrial fibrillation. *J Am Coll Cardiol* 49:565–71.

Girola A, Enrini R, Garbetta F, Tufano A & Caviezel F (2001) QT dispersion in uncomplicated human obesity. *Obes Res* 9:71–7.

Iacobellis G (2005) Is obesity a risk factor for atrial fibrillation? *Nat Clin Pract Cardiovasc Med* 2:134–5.

Iacobellis G, Curione M, Di Bona S, Ribaudo MC, Zappaterreno A & Vecci E (2005) Effect of acute hyperinsulinemia on ventricular repolarization in uncomplicated obesity. *Int J Cardiol* 99:161–3.

Kannel WB, Plehn JF & Cupples LA (1988) Cardiac failure and sudden death in the Framingham Study. *Am Heart J* 115:869–75.

Lalani AP, Kanna B, John J, Ferrick KJ, Huber MS & Shapiro LE (2000) Abnormal signal-averaged electrocardiogram (SAECG) in obesity. *Obes Res* 8:20–8.

Papaioannou A, Michaloudis D, Fraidakis O, *et al.* (2003) Effects of weight loss on QT interval in morbidly obese patients. *Obes Surg* 13:869–73.

Pontiroli AE, Pizzocri P, Saibene A, Girola A, Koprivec D & Fragasso G (2004) Left ventricular hypertrophy and QT interval in obesity and in hypertension: effects of weight loss and of normalisation of blood pressure. *Int J Obes Relat Metab Disord* 28:1118–23.

Seyfeli E, Duru M, Kuvandik G, Kaya H & Yalcin F (2006) Effect of obesity on P-wave dispersion and QT dispersion in women. *Int J Obes (Lond)* 30:957–61.

Wang TJ, Parise H, Levy D, *et al.* (2004) Obesity and the risk of new-onset atrial fibrillation. *JAMA* 292:2471–7.

Wolf J, Lewicka J & Narkiewicz K (2007) Obstructive sleep apnea: an update on mechanisms and cardiovascular consequences. *Nutr Metab Cardiovasc Dis* 17:233–40.

Zacharias A, Schwann TA, Riordan CJ, Durham SJ, Shah AS & Habib RH (2005) Obesity and risk of new-onset atrial fibrillation after cardiac surgery. *Circulation* 112:3247–55.

Weight-loss strategies

Ashrafian H, le Roux CW, Darzi A & Athanasiou T (2008) Effects of bariatric surgery on cardiovascular function. *Circulation* 118:2091–102.

Batsis JA, Romero-Corral A, Collazo-Clavell ML, *et al.* (2007) Effect of weight loss on predicted cardiovascular risk: change in cardiac risk after bariatric surgery. *Obesity (Silver Spring)* 15:772–84.

Belza A, Frandsen E & Kondrup J (2007) Body fat loss achieved by stimulation of thermogenesis by a combination of bioactive food ingredients: a placebo-controlled, double-blind 8-week intervention in obese subjects. *Int J Obes (Lond)* 31:121–30.

Bensimhon DR, Kraus WE & Donahue MP (2006) Obesity and physical activity: a review. *Am Heart J* 151:598–603.

Busetto L, Tregnaghi A, Bussolotto M, *et al.* (2000) Visceral fat loss evaluated by total body magnetic resonance imaging in obese women operated with laparascopic adjustable silicone gastric banding. *Int J Obes Relat Metab Disord* 24:60–9.

Caruso MK, Pekarovic S, Raum WJ & Greenway F (2007) Topical fat reduction from the waist. *Diabetes Obes Metab* 9:300–3.

Cussler EC, Teixeira PJ, Going SB, *et al.* (2008) Maintenance of weight loss in overweight middle-aged women through the Internet. *Obesity (Silver Spring)* 16:1052–60.

Dagenais GR, Yi Q, Mann JF, Bosch J, Pogue J & Yusuf S (2005) Prognostic impact of body weight and abdominal obesity in women and men with cardiovascular disease. *Am Heart J* 149:54–60.

Dapri G, Vaz C, Cadiere GB & Himpens J (2007) A prospective randomized study comparing two different techniques for laparoscopic sleeve gastrectomy. *Obes Surg* 17:1435–41.

Derosa G, Cicero AF, Murdolo G, *et al.* (2005) Efficacy and safety comparative evaluation of orlistat and sibutramine treatment in hypertensive obese patients. *Diabetes Obes Metab* 7:47–55.

Despres JP, Golay A, Sjostrom L & the Rimonabant in Obesity-Lipids Study Group (2005) Effects of rimonabant on metabolic risk factors in overweight patients with dyslipidemia. *N Engl J Med* 353:2121–34.

Di Francesco V, Sacco T, Zamboni M, *et al.* (2007) Weight loss and quality of life improvement in obese subjects treated with sibutramine: a double-blind randomized multicenter study. *Ann Nutr Metab* 51:75–81.

Diepvens K, Soenen S, Steijns J, Arnold M & Westerterp-Plantenga M (2007) Long-term effects of consumption of a novel fat emulsion in relation to body-weight management. *Int J Obes (Lond)* 31:942–9.

Donnelly JE, Sullivan DK, Smith BK, *et al.* (2008) Alteration of dietary fat intake to prevent weight gain: Jayhawk Observed Eating Trial. *Obesity (Silver Spring)* 16:107–12.

Douketis JD & Sharma AM (2005) Obesity and cardiovascular disease: pathogenic mechanisms and potential benefits of weight reduction. *Semin Vasc Med* 5:25–33.

Franz MJ, VanWormer JJ, Crain AL, *et al.* (2007) Weight-loss outcomes: a systematic review and meta-analysis of weight-loss clinical trials with a minimum 1-year follow-up. *J Am Diet Assoc* 107:1755–67.

Ikonomidis I, Mazarakis A, Papadopoulos C, *et al.* (2007) Weight loss after bariatric surgery improves aortic elastic properties and left ventricular function in individuals with morbid obesity: a 3-year follow-up study. *J Hypertens* 25:439–47.

Ilanne-Parikka P, Eriksson JG, Lindstrom J, *et al.* (2008) Effect of lifestyle intervention on the occurrence of metabolic syndrome and its components in the Finnish Diabetes Prevention Study. *Diabetes Care* 31:805–7.

Imaz I, Martinez-Cervell C, Garcia-Alvarez EE, Sendra-Gutierrez JM & Gonzalez-Enriquez J (2008) Safety and effectiveness of the intragastric balloon for obesity. A meta-analysis. *Obes Surg* 18:841–6.

Jakicic JM, Marcus BH, Lang W & Janney C (2008) Effect of exercise on 24-month weight loss maintenance in overweight women. *Arch Intern Med* 168:1550–9; discussion 1559–60.

James WP, Astrup A, Finer N, *et al.* (2000) Effect of sibutramine on weight maintenance after weight loss: a randomised trial. STORM Study Group. Sibutramine Trial of Obesity Reduction and Maintenance. *Lancet* 356:2119–25.

Jones M, Luce KH, Osborne MI, *et al.* (2008) Randomized, controlled trial of an internet-facilitated intervention for reducing binge eating and overweight in adolescents. *Pediatrics* 121:453–62.

Karamanakos SN, Vagenas K, Kalfarentzos F & Alexandrides TK (2008) Weight loss, appetite suppression, and changes in fasting and postprandial ghrelin and peptide-YY levels after Roux-en-Y gastric bypass and sleeve gastrectomy: a prospective, double blind study. *Ann Surg* 247:401–7.

Lubrano C, Cornoldi A, Pili M, *et al.* (2004) Reduction of risk factors for cardiovascular diseases in morbid-obese patients following biliary-intestinal bypass: 3 years' follow-up. *Int J Obes Relat Metab Disord* 28:1600–6.

Maggioni AP, Caterson I, Coutinho W, *et al.* (2008) Tolerability of sibutramine during a 6-week treatment period in high-risk patients with cardiovascular disease and/or diabetes: a preliminary analysis of the Sibutramine Cardiovascular Outcomes (SCOUT) Trial. *J Cardiovasc Pharmacol* 52:393–402.

McGovern L, Johnson JN, Paulo R, *et al.* (2008) Treatment of pediatric obesity. A systematic review and meta-analysis of randomized trials. *J Clin Endocrinol Metab* 93:4600–5.

McMahon FG, Fujioka K, Singh BN, *et al.* (2000) Efficacy and safety of sibutramine in obese white and African American patients with hypertension: a 1-year, double-blind, placebo-controlled, multicenter trial. *Arch Intern Med* 160:2185–91.

McMahon FG, Weinstein SP, Rowe E, *et al.* (2002) Sibutramine is safe and effective for weight loss in obese patients whose hypertension is well controlled with angiotensin-converting enzyme inhibitors. *J Hum Hypertens* 16:5–11.

Nissen SE, Nicholls SJ, Wolski K, *et al.* (2008) Effect of rimonabant on progression of atherosclerosis in patients with abdominal obesity and coronary artery disease: the STRADIVARIUS randomized controlled trial. *JAMA* 299:1547–60.

Okauchi Y, Nishizawa H, Funahashi T, *et al.* (2007) Reduction of visceral fat is associated with decrease in the number of metabolic risk factors in Japanese men. *Diabetes Care* 30:2392–4.

Paineau DL, Beaufils F, Boulier A, *et al.* (2008) Family dietary coaching to improve nutritional intakes and body weight control: a randomized controlled trial. *Arch Pediatr Adolesc Med* 162:34–43.

Pi-Sunyer FX, Aronne LJ, Heshmati HM, Devin J, Rosenstock J & the RIO-North America Study Group (2006) Effect of rimonabant, a cannabinoid-1 receptor blocker, on weight and cardiometabolic risk factors in overweight or obese patients: RIO-North America: a randomized controlled trial. *JAMA* 295:761–75.

Richardson CR, Newton TL, Abraham JJ, Sen A, Jimbo M, Swartz AM (2008) A meta-analysis of pedometer-based walking interventions and weight loss. *Ann Fam Med* 6:69–77.

Shai I, Schwarzfuchs D, Henkin Y, *et al.* (2008) Weight loss with a low-carbohydrate, Mediterranean, or low-fat diet. *N Engl J Med* 359:229–41.

Sharma AM (2001) Sibutramine in overweight/obese hypertensive patients. *Int J Obes Relat Metab Disord* 25 (Suppl. 4):S20–3.

Sharma AM, Caterson ID, Coutinho W, *et al.* (2008) Blood pressure changes associated with sibutramine and weight management—an analysis from the 6-week lead-in period of the sibutramine cardiovascular outcomes trial (SCOUT). *Diabetes Obes Metab* 11:239–50.

Shechter M, Beigel R, Freimark D, Matetzky S & Feinberg MS (2006) Short-term sibutramine therapy is associated with weight loss and improved endothelial function in obese patients with coronary artery disease. *Am J Cardiol* 97:1650–3.

Sjostrom L, Lindroos AK, Peltonen M, *et al.* (2004) Lifestyle, diabetes, and cardiovascular risk factors 10 years after bariatric surgery. *N Engl J Med* 351:2683–93.

Svendsen M, Rissanen A, Richelsen B, Rossner S, Hansson F & Tonstad S (2008) Effect of orlistat on eating behavior among participants in a 3-year weight maintenance trial. *Obesity (Silver Spring)* 16:327–33.

Svetkey LP, Stevens VJ, Brantley PJ, *et al.* (2008) Comparison of strategies for sustaining weight loss: the weight loss maintenance randomized controlled trial. *JAMA* 299:1139–48.

Torp-Pedersen C, Caterson I, Coutinho W, *et al.* (2007) Cardiovascular responses to weight management and sibutramine in high-risk subjects: an analysis from the SCOUT trial. *Eur Heart J* 28:2915–23.

Torquati A, Wright K, Melvin W & Richards W (2007) Effect of gastric bypass operation on Framingham and actual risk of cardiovascular events in class II to III obesity. *J Am Coll Surg* 204:776–82.

Vogel JA, Franklin BA, Zalesin KC, *et al.* (2007) Reduction in predicted coronary heart disease risk after substantial weight reduction after bariatric surgery. *Am J Cardiol* 99:222–6.

Watras AC, Buchholz AC, Close RN, Zhang Z & Schoeller DA (2007) The role of conjugated linoleic acid in reducing body fat and preventing holiday weight gain. *Int J Obes (Lond)* 31:481–7.

Whigham LD, Watras AC & Schoeller DA (2007) Efficacy of conjugated linoleic acid for reducing fat mass: a meta-analysis in humans. *Am J Clin Nutr* 85:1203–11.

Willens HJ, Byers P, Chirinos JA, Labrador E, Hare JM & de Marchena E (2007) Effects of weight loss after bariatric surgery on epicardial fat measured using echocardiography. *Am J Cardiol* 99:1242–5.

Wirth A, Scholze J, Sharma AM, Matiba B & Boenner G (2006) Reduced left ventricular mass after treatment of obese patients with sibutramine: an echocardiographic multicentre study. *Diabetes Obes Metab* 8:674–81.

Index

Please note that page references relating to non-textual content such as Boxes, Figures or Tables are in *italic* print